To
Govern
Evolution

HARCOURT
BRACE
JOVANOVICH
PUBLISHERS
Boston   San Diego   New York

To
Govern
Evolution

FURTHER
ADVENTURES
OF THE
POLITICAL
ANIMAL

Walter
Truett
Anderson

Library of Congress Cataloging in Publication Data

Anderson, Walter Truett.
To govern evolution.

Bibliography: p.
I. Biopolitics. I. Title.
JA80.A53 1986   320'.01'574   86-19477
ISBN 0-15-190483-9

Designed by Michael Farmer
Printed in the United States of America
First Edition
A B C D E

For Mauriça and Dan
with love and hope

It is as if man had been suddenly appointed managing director of the biggest business of all, the business of evolution—appointed without being asked if he wanted it, and without proper warning and preparation. What is more, he can't refuse the job. Whether he wants it or not, whether he is conscious of what he is doing or not, he is in point of fact determining the future direction of evolution on this earth. That is his inescapable destiny, and the sooner he realizes it and starts believing in it, the better for all concerned.

—*Julian Huxley*

People have forgotten this truth, but you must not forget it. You become responsible forever, for what you have tamed. You are responsible for your rose.

—*Antoine de Saint-Exupéry*

[Contents]

[Preface]

JOSEPH CONRAD made a comment about writing that I thought of often as I was working on this book. Conrad said: "My task which I am trying to achieve is, by the power of the written word to make you hear, to make you feel—it is, before all, to make you *see.*" He was speaking of the craft of fiction, of course; one might be more inclined to say of nonfiction that the writer's task is to persuade, to inform—with luck, to interest—the reader. But I find as I have worked on this book that the thing I most want to say to the reader is: "Look." Look at this. Look at that. Look at these things grouped together. Much of what follows is my attempt to direct your attention to certain features of the political landscape, to get you to observe the confluence of certain events. This book is, before all, an effort at creating a perspective.

The best I can do to describe that perspective in a preliminary way, for the reader who wants a sense of where we are going, is to say that it has to do with the connections between biology and politics, between nature and humanity.

A word like "connections" is not quite right, however, because it implies that there is some preexisting separation between biology and politics, between nature and humanity, and that our task is to forge links among them. Our task is more difficult than that—it is to discover their inseparability.

There is much talk these days, as people encounter the new wonders of the Biological Revolution, about the need for humanity to learn to live within nature. I sympathize with the sentiment, but unfortunately such statements are quite meaningless. They can have no meaning unless they are supported by some clear idea of a difference between living in nature and living in non-nature. And since we do not (and *can* not) have any such clear idea, discussion of the most important issues of our time bogs down before it can even begin, and well-meant searches for value slide quickly into cant and empty rhetoric.

This problem is serious, but not insurmountable. It can be resolved by some thinking about how people have interacted with nature (and how they have thought about it), and it can be resolved by some looking.

So I will invite you to look—literally—at your personal environment, and will suggest that it has much information to communicate. Beyond that I will ask you to consider some events in the planet's history, and a few things that are now going on in the biosphere—not the least important of which is the emergence of an idea of a biosphere.

All this is preparation for forming a perspective about human power in nature.

Human power in nature is the ultimate political issue, and it is easy to take an unexamined stance in regard to it. One such position would be to say there should not be any such power, that human beings should not intervene in nature at all. This is an admirable principle in the abstract, but since no human society practices it—not even the most primitive or most reverent—it is of no value whatever as a guideline for modern life. A step more satisfactory is the answer that we should practice ecology. This is quite true—the time will come when governance and ecology are understood to be more or less the same thing—but for "ecology" to be used with any meaning requires some idea of what the ecosystems we inhabit really are, how they work, and how they are changing. That reality, as I will attempt to show you, is considerably different from the image most of us call up in our minds when the word "ecosystem" is used.

The environment is the base from which we think and act as political beings. The more accurate our understanding of it, the more effective our ideas and actions are likely to be; we have to know the territory.

We are entering a new political territory, and new political issues are emerging in it. I will not attempt to conceal my own opinions about those issues or refrain from advocating courses of action, but it is not my purpose—not in this work, at least—to develop an ideology or put forth a set of policy recommendations. I am sure that many sensible ideas and policies will come forth if we can get our attention directed toward the right issues. The famous political boss Ed Flynn used to say that he didn't care who did the electing as long as he could do the nominating—and in a similar vein I think the real power in the realm of public dialogue lies not so much in influencing opinions as in influencing what it is that people believe they need to have opinions about. If I can get you to form opinions about some of the issues raised in these pages, I will consider my time well spent.

A final word about the field of vision. The perspective I wish to develop is a global one, and yet I will approach evolution as a concept developed within Western civilization, cite events in European history and American politics, and often discuss issues current in the state and region in which I live. I am aware that there are inherent limitations in this, that these matters might be approached in a very different way by someone living in another part of the world and educated to a different history—yet it is my belief that, wherever we start from, we come to the point where histories and cultures converge. So I view the biosphere from my own place in it—literally from my own back yard, as you will see in Chapter One—and leave my tracks uncovered as I proceed in search of universals.

In the years since I began this work I have had many occasions to discuss it and the ideas in it with different groups of friends and colleagues—a local writers' circle, another group that meets monthly for dinner and conversation, the weekly idea meetings at Pacific News Service and an annual conference on governance. I cannot mention here all the names of all the people who have participated in these rites, but I would like to acknowledge, in an anonymous *en masse* blessing, how rich and valuable to me that kind of dialogue has been.

Among those who have read the manuscript at various stages of its life and/or provided information, ideas, criticism and encouragement are William Adams, Jack Ballard, John Berger, Clem Bezold, Richard Boeke, Lynton Caldwell, Ernest Callenbach, Fritjof Capra, Sandy Close, Jack and Jeff Fobes, Richard Grossman, Rasa Gustaitis, Mary Gardiner Jones, Doug Lea, Abe Levitsky, Don Michael, Brian Murphy, Jay Ogilvy, Robert Olson, Pat Ophuls, Hink and Elsa Porter, Houston Smith, Charlene Spretnak,

Richard Register, Ted Roszak, Franz Schurmann, Keith Thompson, Jürgen Voigt, Steve Waldhorn, Tom Wilson and Burke Zimmerman. I especially want to acknowledge my intellectual debt to Don Michael, whose thoughts on learning, planning and governance are evident in many places here; and to Rollo May, whose ideas regarding power and innocence are far more influential on my own than the one citation in Chapter Nine would indicate. And, finally, my gratitude to my own family, Dan and both Mauriças, for the powerful affirmation that comes from simply letting me know that whatever I want to do is all right with them. I suspect that only other writers will know how important this is.

To
Govern
Evolution

[I]

The Political
Econiche

THE CENTRAL political problem of our time is not that people in power do the wrong things, or that some people have more power than others, or that there is a lack of clarity and honesty in political dialogue; all of these are real and serious, but they are only dim reflections of a larger problem, which is that we literally do not know what we are doing. We have no concept of what politics is about that fits the reality of the present situation. Even though the air is thick with talk of paradigm shifts and predictions of a new global post-industrial civilization, we seem unable—or afraid—to grasp the truth of how the world has changed, and what it means to govern.

This truth is both highly complex and quite simple: Politics is about evolution. Governance is inextricably connected with the growing human responsibility for all the things the word "evolution" implies: the survival and extinction of species, the changing ecology of the planet, the biological (and cultural) condition of the human species itself. Evolution no longer follows the Darwinian rules that provided, for over a century, our best understanding of it. It is no longer an impersonal and mechanistic process obeying the remorseless logic of natural selection. That vision is as obsolete as its first cousin, Newton's clockwork cosmos. Today the driving force in evolution is human intelligence. Species survive or perish because of what people do to them and to their environments. The land and air and water systems are massively altered by humankind which has become, as one scientist put it, "a new geological force." Even our own genetic future is in our hands, guided not by Darwinian abstractions but by science and medical technology and public policy. The world has changed; and the human species, which has wrought the change, is now being required to change in response to conditions we have created.

The change calls for a massive reappraisal of basic ideas. Old definitions no longer serve as well as they once did, and barriers crumble between compartments of thought. We have conceived of politics and evolution as two different things, not quite in the same category of meaning, no more to be added together than the proverbial apples and oranges. We have taken politics to consist of interactions among human beings. The word politics comes from the Greek *polis*, which meant both city and state; it evokes an image of human beings jostling in the marketplace, worshipping in the temple, competing for influence and power. We have a corresponding ideal of government of the *people*, by the *people*, for the *people*. Evolution, on the other hand, has to do with nature, with plants and animals and their environments, with a grand sweep of change that proceeds according to laws beyond human reach. That is how we think of the two—and that is the

[2]

problem, because the two are now one. They have flowed together, and there is no making sense of one without reference to the other.

I am not here to argue that the human species ought to take responsibility for evolution on the planet, and begin through public and private institutions to make collective decisions about such matters. If that were the question to be decided I would advocate that we put it off for a few centuries or more—let things run themselves while we get accustomed to the idea of evolutionary governance, develop the appropriate ethics and myths and political structures, and perhaps mature a bit. However, that is not the question before us, since we are already governing evolution. This is the great paradox about the threshold: It is not out there ahead of us somewhere, a line from which we might conceivably draw back. We are well across it. To say that we are not ready for evolutionary governance is equivalent to saying that a teenage child is not ready for puberty; the statement may be true, but it is not much help.

Every era in history has its own master challenge, a central problem or project that dominates the times. Paul Tillich writes that the preoccupation of the classical Greek era was the mind's search for the eternal Immovable, while the Middle Ages were dominated by the attempt to create a social and political order within the framework of Christian faith.[1] Recent centuries have been given over to the projects of science and industry—increasing human understanding of the natural universe and devising new modes of productivity. We are now moving into an age which will be dominated by the discovery that science and industry, by achieving an unprecedented degree of human power over the workings of nature, have created an entirely new order of problems and presented us with a new overriding project. We will be required to come to terms with the reality of ever-growing human ability to intervene in nature. We will have to recognize that human power has increased to an extent that transforms both human society and the biosphere, and makes of the two a *de facto* unit. We will have to understand that the use of this power is in essence a political challenge.

Because the theme of this book—evolutionary governance—is an unfamiliar one, I want to make my argument as accessible as possible to the reader. In order to do this, I offer three basic assertions about this power/biosphere challenge: A prediction about the future, a statement about the present, and a statement about the past. I will try to make these clear and straightforward so that the reader may consider them, weigh them against any available evidence, and accept or reject them accordingly.

The prediction about the future: The decades ahead will be dominated by the Biological Revolution, in which a cascade of scientific and technological developments will significantly (and *continually*, with ongoing innovation and escalating rates of change) increase human ability to intervene in nature. This wave of change will compel us to modify some of our most basic biological concepts (parenthood, for example) and will alter the conditions of life for all people everywhere. This will be a traumatic development in many ways and will produce both great benefits and serious social and personal disruptions. I have yielded in a couple of previous writings to the temptation to describe it as "bioshock". The potential of the Biological Revolution has been seriously underrated by most futurists, and there is a good reason for this: You cannot make out the shape of the future if you do not know where you

[4]

are in the present. This brings me to my second point, the statement about the present:

We are now in the midst of a large-scale alteration of the biosphere, which is partly the result of historical processes that have been underway for centuries, and partly the product of the myriad economic, scientific and technological forces of modern society. At the global level this alteration is identifiable by such events as the rapid extinction of species and a kind of homogenization of ecosystems around the world as plants and animals are moved from one place to another. At the level of personal and family life it is marked by the appearance of new technologies of birth control, genetic screening and reproduction which alter the rules of human birth; and by new medical technologies which alter the rules of human life and death. We do not inhabit the same kind of a biosphere that people of only a generation past inhabited, and we are not the same kind of biological beings that our parents were.

The statement about the past: People have consistently misread (or ignored) the evidence about their interventions in nature. Just as a misreading of the biopolitical present renders us vulnerable to failing to foresee future developments, so does a misreading of history dim our awareness of what kind of a world we are living in today.

If we are indeed already in an era of evolutionary governance, we must have been heading in this direction for some time. Such transitions do not happen in an instant. And in fact this one has been stealing upon us for tens of thousands of years, unseen largely because we did not want to see it. No single event marks the point at which the human species became responsible for global evolution; rather, human history and prehistory have been crowded with such events, and each event has served to make the pattern more clear, the general tendency less reversible. The responsibility increases, and it increases with accelerating speed. One might single out among the more recent markers of the trend such events as the Industrial Revolution, the more recent mechanization of agriculture, the series of advances in hygiene and immunology and medicine which stimulated increases in the rate of human population growth, and the emergence of the science of genetics in this century. I would choose as the most important single event the publication of *The Origin of Species*. It brought an end to the long era in which people had seen the world as a stable and unchanging natural order, and gave rise to a new world-view of ongoing creation and change. It also opened an era of discovery—one that is still going on—in which the genetic processes that shape evolutionary change are comprehended in ever-greater detail.

Power in Nature

I SAID earlier that the Darwinian laws have been repealed, and here I assert that *The Origin of Species* opened the door to the present era. This sounds contradictory, yet it is quite obvious from the historical record that Darwin's work was a major contributor to its own obsolescence. As soon as the human species accepted the proposition that nature changes, it moved rapidly toward further discoveries which enabled people to influence such change far more effectively than they had in the past. Darwin thought it was possible for human beings to stand apart from the world of nature and comprehend its principles without intervening in the processes involved. It is now

[6]

apparent, however, that the realm of nature Darwin described, the one serenely evolving according to the rules of natural selection, no longer exists. Scientific discoveries—in the life sciences, in geology and chemistry and physics—move rapidly from theory to application, merge with other lines of human endeavor, and re-shape the world along the way. We underestimate the extent of such changes, do not comprehend that in a sense there is no "nature" left in the world. Sometimes, in discussions of this subject, I ask someone to identify a place in the world that can be called completely and pristinely "natural" in contrast to places—such as, say, Central Park—which are obviously creations of human artifice. And as we do so we find that no absolute distinction can be made; we find that a set of definitions that are universally used and taken to be simple truth have no real operational meaning. There is no place on Earth—certainly not on an Earth whose sunlight filters through an ozone layer that has been accidentally altered by human technology—that is truly, as the saying goes, untouched by human hands. Indeed, all the things we do to preserve "nature", everything from wilderness management to endangered species legislation, are in one way or another human interventions.

The transition we are talking about here is a whole-system transition—not merely a transition or turning-point in human history, but a transition in the evolution of the planet itself.

Our ways of talking about this are rough-hewn; such a transition has not happened before and we have nothing to compare it with. We might be in a much different position if we had been able to gather any data on the growth and maturation of planets that had developed intelligent life. If we had information about a few thousand such planets—or even about one besides our own—we might have a concept of patterns of development with recognizeable stages. This would be somewhat similar to what we find in the work of psychologists like Piaget and Erickson, who have identified phases that people pass through as they move from infancy to old age. A human being is a marvelously complex organism, and its growth has many dimensions. Each transition changes the chemistry of the body, the personality, the self-concept, the individual's morality or code of ethics. A planet's stages would be seen as even more complex, and a "turning point" might take hundreds or even thousands of years. The appearance of life on Earth was one such turning point, and the discovery by one living species of the principles of evolution is another.

As human knowledge and power increase, the rules change for all living things on the planet. Plants and animals that have endured for millennia now live in a different world, a world they never made, and their survival as individuals or as species is determined not only by their own adaptive skills, but by the things people do to preserve them or render them extinct—and also by what is sometimes called the "Lilliput effect", the repercussions of distant, sometimes accidental or careless human actions. DDT's history provides a good example of the Lilliput effect: DDT did what was expected of it—was an effective weapon against mosquitoes, dramatically reduced malaria in many regions—and it also had a host of unexpected side effects. In some areas it killed off predatory insects which were DDT-vulnerable and produced massive increases in the populations of other pests (such as spider mites) which were DDT-resistant. It caused birds to lay eggs with thinner shells, thereby jeopardizing the survival of several species. It spread through food chains until it became detectable in the fatty tissue of Northern Eskimos and Antarctic penguins and seals, and in human milk. The use of DDT is in fact an intervention in evolution, improving the survival prospects for some life forms and reducing them for others. Its impacts are on a global scale, and the species it affects number in the thousands. Many such Lilliput effects reverberate now about the globe, and nothing that lives is isolated from them.

We have made the transition into *acts* of evolutionary governance, but we have not yet developed a *concept* of evolutionary governance. What we call the modern age has been a kind of "window"—to borrow a term from the defense strategists—between the time when a burst of scientific discoveries and technological developments brought an enormous increase in the extent of human intervention in evolutionary processes and the present, when we are forced by the accumulation of a mountain of evidence to recognize what we are doing. This is the project of the coming era: to create a social and political order—a global one—commensurate to human power in nature. The project requires a shift from evolutionary meddling to evolutionary governance, informed by an ethic of responsibility—an evolutionary ethic, not merely an environmental ethic—and it requires appropriate ways of thinking about new issues and making decisions. It involves public policy; matters of survival and extinction are already being legislated everywhere. It involves political philosophy; old ideologies will metamorphose, and new ones will emerge. It involves a general recognition, one that will have to be articulated throughout human society, that the human species has developed a specialized role in the global ecosystem. It also presents an opportunity to define humanity itself in a new way, to bring new meaning into our private and political life.

The existential philosophers—particularly Sartre—used to lament that humanity lacked an essential purpose, had been thrown willy-nilly into the cosmos and condemned to find whatever order it could in life while walking always along the brink of utter meaninglessness. This was a bleak perspective in many ways, but it had a courageous side to it: It spoke for intentionality, for individual life as a mighty struggle to impose personal meaning on existential chaos.

We find now that the human predicament is not quite so devoid of inherent purpose after all. To be caretakers of a planet, custodians of all its life forms and shapers of its (and our own) future is certainly purpose enough. It is a challenge furthermore, with all the trappings of high adventure. It brings danger and mystery, it calls for cleverness and courage, and it promises great rewards. We do not have any choice, now, about whether or not to accept this challenge. Our ancestors have been unwittingly preparing the stage for us from the time they began walking upright, have altered the world in so many ways that now even our attempts at preservation are further alterations.

We have told ourselves this kind of story many times. In myths and legends and fairy tales and adventure stories— in the places where the circuitous human mind hides the things it doesn't much want to know but can't quite afford to forget—the tale of the reluctant hero recurs again and again. Bilbo Baggins in the J.R.R. Tolkien books is a recent example: Bilbo is not a *macho* hero at all, merely a quiet home-loving hobbit who wants to be comfortable and enjoy himself, and who dislikes adventures because they make you late for dinner. But he is swept away by forces beyond himself (although we are given to suspect that he may be more willing than he admits) and is off on a vast journey into the unknown.

There is a similar kind of destiny in human existence, an evolutionary story in which we have a certain role to play and no option to refuse. This hardly means that the element of choice and freedom disappears from our lives. On the contrary, the choices are here in abundance. As a polis, we legislate the survival or extinction of species, manage the atmosphere. As individuals, we can choose how many children we have, are increasingly capable of basing such choices on advance knowledge of the genetic characteristics of unborn children, and are not far from being able to pre-choose the sex of a child. The present state of nuclear arms stockpiling gives the human species the ultimate choice of biocide, the end of all life on the planet. It is our lot to fret about such choices, and our lot to have them. They are indicators of the human econiche.

Every species occupies an econiche, which is a way of saying that it has a certain role, a relationship to other species in the same ecosystem. The human species, by virtue of its present level of evolution, has a relationship to all species in all ecosystems. This is an essential part of the transition: One species on the planet, and one species only, has reached the point of being able to have an impact on the evolutionary fortunes of all other species and upon the functioning of all ecosystems. We also have, in a way that is not true for any other species, a relationship to the planet as a whole and to the future. We live with all life.

This truth defines us collectively, in a way that no previous biological classification of the human species has ever done, and it applies to each individual human being. To be a member of a species that has reached such an evolutionary point is to be required to go through the daily business of life with a different sense of connection and purpose. And our situation also alters the basic conditions of our political existence.

The New Polis

ARISTOTLE, in a definition of the human species that has held up well for over two thousand years, said that we are the political animal—that the human being is truly human only in society and not only in society but in the polis, the social order that is created out of human volition.

People do not feel comfortable knowing that the polis is a human creation and have a hankering to be back in the Garden with the rest of animal life, living within social orders encoded in the genes. We pretend that our states were created by God or by superhuman lawgivers. We create about the state an aura of sanctity that makes it seem to have some existence of its own, and preserve the structures of states long after the circumstances that gave rise to them have disappeared. This is not an entirely bad idea—revolutions make you late for dinner too—but it lets us forget that even when we choose to retain the systems we have, even when we try to make no choice at all and merely support a system passively by doing nothing to change it, we are being political in a way that is not available to an elephant or a bee.

Considering how nervous we are about knowing that the human species creates its institutional environment, it is hardly surprising that we avoid knowing that we create our "natural" environments as well, make up our ecosystems. Yet that is the truth the times force upon us, the one that every generation before ours has managed to avoid. They desired to avoid it because it carried responsibilities, and they were able to avoid it because there was always more room somewhere, because there were not too many people, because energy and resources and food still appeared to be unlimited, because science and technology were less lethal, because pollution disappeared, because scientists had not yet started tinkering with DNA molecules. We could pretend that our actions on the Earth were benign and limited—that we only made a few improvements here, practiced a little domestication and cultivation there. But now the evidence crowds all around us; we are obliged to know what we do in the world, to see that it has changed and that we are the makers of the change.

Once we see that there is no untouched nature, that the environments in which we live—not only our homes and gardens, but our continents—are human artifacts, we are in a position to awaken to the reality of the change.

One way to approach this concept is through history. That was the path along which I first approached it—or, to be more accurate, along which it first approached me. The outlines of the perspective from which this book is written took shape during the writing of an earlier book, *A Place of Power: The American Episode in Human Evolution*, which was published in 1976. That started out to be a more or less conventional text on American government, but as I researched the historical background I became strongly drawn to the details of what is usually called "natural history". I considered the "clearing away" of forest that was part of every colonist's work, the endless battle of the American farmer against weeds and predators, and the massive importation of new species from other parts of the world—everything from insects to apple trees. The single discovery that intrigued me the most was that the Mayflower's passengers included not only those human pilgrims so well remembered in the history books and the social registers, but also pigs and sheep and cattle, and smaller pilgrims—like dandelions in the food larders and moths in the woolen clothes. I found new significance in something whose import had slipped by me in earlier forays into American history—the extensive program of "internal improvements" that the new federal government undertook in the first years of the Washington administration: cutting interstate canals, dredging coastal harbors, laying out high roads through the fields and forests. I had known that the colonists came from Europe, and took the land. I had known that they established a new form of government upon it, created a polis. But I had not known that they systematically—with a consensus so strong it never even needed to be articulated, much less debated—rebuilt the American continent into something more suitable to their purposes, something suspiciously similar to the European continent they had left. The story resembled a science-fiction saga of people coming to a planet and gradually converting it. I quoted Woody Guthrie's song "This Land Was Made for You and Me," which now took on an entirely new load of meaning, and wrote:

> The whole thrust and purpose of the American experience has been in the direction of (1) bringing to this continent a vast number of people from other parts of the world, and (2) modifying this continent to make it suitable for the kind of social organization its new inhabitants wanted. Over the rather brief span of centuries

that American history covers, we have built a huge, artificial ecosystem of farms and factories and cities, artificial waterways and sculptured land spaces. This is what we must now run—and keep it running, because it sustains our lives.

The American continent has been transformed; it is now an artificial ecosystem and it must be managed by human action. This cannot be stopped, now, nor can we return to a natural order untouched by human society. We are at the controls, whether we like it or not. If suddenly the human race were to disappear from the North American continent there would be a period of ecological chaos followed by the emergence of a new balance of nature. But it would have very little resemblance to the America that existed before Columbus arrived. And since we do not intend to disappear and do not know how to live in anything but an artificial ecosystem, we would do well to confront the fact that we have indeed created one and now must manage it. We must confront the fact that our "system"—the whole political/social/economic interaction—must govern the entire physical space of America, all its water and air and living creatures.

When the new political system we now call the United States of America was organized and put into operation, it became the legitimate government of its citizens. Following the recognized concept of the nation-state as a territorial entity, it assumed jurisdiction over the physical space itself, the land and water within its borders. Furthermore, it assumed governing power over all the other living creatures within that physical space. American history does not indicate that the birds, beasts, and flowers were ever consulted on this point, but nevertheless their lives came under the control of the new human civilization. There was, of course, no explicit discussion of this dimension of political power at the time. It was an implicit and unquestioned part of the consciousness of Western culture, as old as Genesis.[2]

A Place of Power was a book about American history and American natural history (two phrases we use for what is really one subject) and it becomes apparent now that the American experience, the biological conquest of the continent, was different only in certain details (chiefly time scale) from a larger, indeed world-wide, process. The American saga of colonists and pioneers is only a dramatic foreshortening of what has happened everywhere, as human beings wrought artifical ecosystems out of the rough clay of their environments. In this respect, as in some others, American history is human history in the large print edition. The whole world is an artificial ecosystem.

History is an excellent path along which to travel toward an understanding of the human econiche. If we all knew our American natural history—the truth symbolized by Paul Bunyan and Johnny Appleseed—we would stand on firmer ground in regard to the present and the future. But history is not the only source. The truth is as close as the nearest window. Out there is a segment of your environment, the water in which you are a fish. It is said that a fish does not know it is in water, does not see the major component of its ecosystem. What we look at but rarely see is the artificiality that surrounds us. We may see it if the view is of buildings and paved streets; we may be less likely to see it if we look out at plants and animals—it takes a bit of reflection to see how many of them are hybrids and inventions, imports and invaders, brought here by human action and maintained by human action.

In California, where I live, modification of the environment accelerated with the arrival of the first explorers and settlers from Europe. In the eighteenth century, 20 million acres of California lowlands were fields of tall grasses. Then the Spaniards came, inadvertently bringing new seeds with them—perhaps in the wool of sheep, perhaps in hay stored aboard ships for livestock. These European invaders proved hardier than the native varieties, and the tall bunch grasses were replaced by the short grasses and thistles. The pace of change increased again with the Gold Rush; new people arrived by the thousands, scrambled through the mountains and foothills, dug in the ground and diverted the rivers, washed away tons of earth with hydraulic mining devices, hunted some species of the native wildlife to extinction. The population increase spurred the demand for new food supplies; soon herds of sheep and cattle were grazing on the land, and there are few ecosystem-transformers to equal a herd of sheep. Farming started on a small scale and expanded quickly to agribusiness. Frank Norris' California novel *The Octopus* describes a scene on a large corporate land holding in the 1870s when thirty-five gang plows were driven like a column of field artillery across the San Joaquin Valley, cutting one hundred and seventy-five simultaneous furrows in the soil. (Any conservationist who had been present to watch the wheat crops displace the European grasses might have thought he or she was witnessing the destruction of the natural environment; one person's modified ecosystem is another's nature.)

California had its wheat booms and its cotton booms, and other long-forgotten flurries of experimentation: A silk boom, intended to make California the silk center of the world, brought into the state shiploads of silkworms and mulberry trees. A eucalyptus boom in the early 1900s produced no more instant millionaires than the silk boom had, but it left the land populated with tall trees from Australia. Forests were cleared, swamps drained, deserts irrigated, dams and canals built to transport water to farms and cities. Native plants and animals perished, and new ones came to take their places: Herefords, Jerseys, and Holsteins; Rhode Island Reds and Poland-China hogs; German brown trout to stock the fishing streams; cats and dogs to roam the streets; vegetables from many parts of the world; orange trees from China and, from Asia Minor, palm trees to start the date orchards and line the streets of Beverly Hills. In the process the land changed and changed again, and today naturalists argue among themselves about what California was like two hundred years ago and perform clever feats of detective work (such as analyzing the grass used in mud bricks from ancient adobes) to reconstruct the not-too-distant past.[3]

From the window of my office, in a house near the eastern shore of the San Francisco Bay, I look out and see many trees, few of them native to this area. Most are immigrants, from Asia and Europe and other parts of North America. Closer, in my patio, are a couple of Italian stone pines in planters and a little evergreen from Washington state that arrived one day at an office where I was working. It came in a pencil-sized tube, as some sort of a promotion for the Great Northwest. It was passed around ("Anybody want this tree?") and I brought it home and it now does well in a pot, somewhat overshadowed by a huge pink dahlia from Germany. In our vegetable garden grow plants native to Central and South America, to the Mediterranean, to Asia; at night the garden snails, descendants of *caracoles* the Spaniards brought for food, come out to munch their leaves. We water our plants regularly; our water comes from Pardee reservoir in the Sierra, about 150 miles away. The air we share with them is fairly clean for an urban area. It is of course monitored by the local Air Pollution Control District, and meets the guidelines set down by the federal clean air legislation: has only moderate quantities of carbon monoxide, oxidants, suspended particulates, ozone, nitrogen dioxide, hydrocarbons, and lead.

From my window I do not see the enormous flocks of geese and ducks that filled these skies not so long ago, the bald eagles and herds of elk and deer. The giant golden bear is now extinct, surviving in Berkeley only as the emblem of the football team. The terrain itself has changed. The San Francisco Bay is about a block farther from here than it used to be, because landfill has reduced its size while expanding the waterfront real estate.

Such is the view from my window. In other places, it is harder to detect the human hand. If you were aboard a ship on the ocean you would have to analyze the water, or count the whales. If you were in the Antarctic you would have to know about the DDT. If you were a hardy frontier person in Alaska you would see only untamed nature, and would probably not think about it much anyway; you would be too busy hacking away at the local flora and fauna, trying to remodel your ecosystem, which is what hardy frontier people do for a living.

As you begin to understand the nature of your environment or, to be more to the point, the non–nature of it, you also begin to understand precisely what kind of an organism you are, how you live and how you will die. You are a political animal in a way that Aristotle never expected a person to be, because the artificial environment you occupy, your personal ecosystem, is a vast and complex network of connections to human beings, human institutions, human laws, human science and technology.

The Ohlone Indians, who once occupied the land where my house now stands, lived their lives within a slightly modified ecosystem, interacting only within small tribal groups. They had no need to interact with people twenty miles away, and very few ever did. Today nobody lives in such simplicity, not even the back-to-nature people who move to the country with their solar collectors and Whole Earth Catalogs. Our bodies are linked by countless arteries and veins and neural pathways to public utilities, government agencies, drug manufacturers, distant growers and packagers of food. We do not inhale or take a drink of water or eat a meal without plugging into a gigantic, increasingly, global web of interconnections among people, organizations, machines and modified ecosystems: the new polis.

This news will come hard to people who would like to believe they are apolitical. The unfortunate truth is that there is no being apolitical in the new polis. You can pretend to drop out of the system, but the system will not drop out of you. The reality of evolutionary governance, of the different world that human beings have created without quite knowing they were doing it, is not only that we have taken responsibility for other species and for the future of the planet, but also that we have hooked ourselves into a monumentally intricate matrix of human interaction. And we are vastly confused about it. We talk about getting government off our backs, and do not notice that it flows in our bloodstreams; we seek self-sufficiency, and in the very attempt to do so enter new forms of interdependence; we defend national sovereignty, and do not perceive that the borders around a nation-state are as quaintly meaningless as the decaying walls that still surround some ancient cities.

We are in new terrain; personal life and political thinking and doing operate under different rules now than they once did and we must, as a first step in any direction, get the feel for the situation. It is one of great choice and possibility, yet also fraught with danger: an adventure, in every sense of the word, and the biggest one that any of us will ever see.

One of the great curiosities of human civilization is that we have moved so far into this terrain without knowing we were doing so. The human urge to avoid that knowledge takes many forms. Environmentalists have one version of avoidance; they are the preeminent good guys of today's drama, but there runs through their green ranks a strong attraction toward a simplified view of our present ecological situation—a perceived split between a realm of nature, which is good, and human action, which is largely bad. Words such as "manage" and "control" provoke nervous responses, suggestions that the proper future scenario for right-thinking people is one in which the human species stops interfering in nature. Evidence that there is no discernable boundary between the human and the natural, that the world has already become a largely artificial and artificially-maintained ecosystem, confuses this agenda. Not long ago, in the course of researching a magazine article about species extinction, I interviewed a young man who worked for a conservationist organization. He showed me a map of "nature preserves" that his organization had helped to establish around the state of California—places where human activity would be restricted and ecological diversity would be preserved. I looked at the map and noted that most of the preserves were in areas that had been extensively modified by various events in California's busy history. "We don't talk about that," he said, and asked me not to mention it in my article. He was right; it is hard enough to get people to contribute money for preserving nature. Getting them to contribute money for maintaining some rough facsimile of natural ecological diversity in a state that has been transformed in a century is a bit too much to ask. Not all environmentalists are still clinging to the back-to-nature creed—a far more sophisticated environmentalism is already evolving—but its poetic appeal and its essential decency make it a powerful, if uninformed, force.

Another type of avoidance of responsibility is the one that a New York Times article some years ago called "the Old-Time Darwin." The writer of this op-ed piece, a corporate PR man, revived the doctrine of survival of the fittest and argued that there was no reason to worry about species becoming extinct. "The Darwin people," he explained, "tell us that species come and go, that this is nature's way of experimenting with life. The successful experiments survive for a time; the failures disappear to no one's detriment."[4] This relaxing idea is expressed frequently, usually with reference to policies for protecting endangered species. Another quite similar refrain is the reminder that there has always been risk and danger in nature, and so it is unreasonable to try to eliminate it by controlling pollution or other such acts of ecological do-gooding. Both these arguments edge away from recognizing that the real issue is human choice. Species no longer become extinct because of failure to adapt to their environments, but because of human impacts on those environments. And we are hardly close to eliminating risk and danger from the world. We have added handsomely to the amount of it: made the water riskier to drink and the air riskier to breathe, invented whole new orders of risk such as the greenhouse effect and nuclear war. The world we live in is shaped by human acts, and the Old-Time Darwin theme, despite its sound of hearty realism, is a fantasy.

The third major route of escape is the Old-Time Religion, which turns out to be surprisingly similar to the Old-Time Darwin in its willingness to lend support to the imperatives of economic progress. The Creationists reject the concept of evolution entirely and read Genesis as the literally true account of how the cosmos came into being and how life emerged on the Earth. Creationists give a nod to the concept of stewardship, but on the whole seem to believe that in practice any responsibility for the Creation is God's rather than their own. Fundamentalist Christianity has its own peculiar form of environmental ethic, admirably expressed in former Secretary of Interior James Watt's celebrated Congressional testimony that, the Second Coming being imminent, long-range concern about environmental matters is not in order and people should make maximum use of resources, as God intended. Secretary Watt did not, of course, speak for all Christianity any more than the back-to-nature troops speak for all environmentalism; we are in a time of ideological upheaval, and there are divisions within every camp.

[23]

Yet it is remarkable that, for all the controversy about such matters, you can find among people of so many different persuasions a common reluctance to recognize and celebrate the full extent of human intervention in the evolutionary process. This reluctance appears in many forms, and its roots go deep into the human psyche and human history.

A BRIEF road map to the material that follows: The next chapter will review a few major points about our evolutionary history, with particular attention to the Darwinian years. Then come four chapters dealing with contemporary issues of evolutionary politics. In the final three chapters, we search for the outlines of a political metamorphosis, and consider ways to move from a present in which a few matters of evolutionary policy are debated among small groups of specialists into a future in which evolution becomes—as it must become—everybody's business.

I have spoken of "problems" and "challenges," but often in the text of the book (and in the title) I refer to adventures. We look at the adventure of moving through a period of global biological instability, the adventure of entering a new stage in human reproductivity, the adventure of stretching our political ideas to accomodate the rights of plants and animals, the adventure of creating a biopolitical culture and a global polis, the adventure of restoring the Earth. I choose the word "adventure" quite deliberately because it is a word that recognizes danger while carrying a banner of enterprise and hope. If the contemplation of the tasks before us is not to be utterly crushing to the human spirit we need to see them in some light that makes them bearable. The world is already overburdened with problems, but we can always use more adventures.

[2]

Toward Evolutionary Governance: A Path of Reluctant Progress

HISTORY HAS been a long march in the direction of increasing human power over the environment and over the evolution of species—but this has been a curious kind of progress, fraught with fear and backward glances, along a path shadowed by self-deception.

Homo sapiens is the only species that evolves reluctantly. From the time our ancestors developed the ability to communicate in symbols—thereby acquiring the makings of a collective past and future, and beginning the process of true human evolution—they appear to have had mixed feelings about whether forward or back was the preferable way to go. Human beings have sometimes created elaborate ideologies of progress and entertained glorious dreams of times to come—and just as often have regarded change as evil and believed that the good old days were gone. We seek knowledge—which is power—and yet shrink from it.

Consider the message of Genesis, one of our greatest myths and a basic underpinning of Judeo-Christian culture.

It is essentially a story of loss, of a falling-away from a condition of idyllic joy. A few verses, as ambiguous and haunting as a Zen landscape, tell of beings who tasted the forbidden fruit of knowledge, and who as a result were cast out of the garden and condemned to exist by tilling the fields and herding flocks in a world where brother turns against brother. Although we usually think of Genesis and evolution as conflicting accounts of the human past, Genesis can also be read as a rich evolutionary parable. It reminds us that the human species feels the transition from its pre-human condition as part gain, part loss. It tells us something we need to understand about the fear of knowing. It shows the acquisition of knowledge as a sin—the original sin—punishable by exile from the garden.

The human attitude toward knowledge is curiously am-bivalent. Intelligence is so predominately what distinguishes the human species from others that we have made it part of our scientific name for ourselves, *Homo sapiens*. We strive incessantly for information about how the cosmos and our own world work, how our minds and bodies work; we sift the ancient soils in search of knowledge about the past and use our shiny new computer technology to try to map out the future. We have amassed a huge amount of knowledge and transformed our lives with it. The contemporary human being lives in a vast open terrain with new vistas in all directions—yet we suffer a collective agoraphobia and look about for someplace to hide our heads. "Strange fate for man!" wrote Samuel Butler. "He must perish if he gets that, which he must perish if he strive not after."[1] Psychologists from Freud onward have commented on the human's mind remarkable ability to erect defenses against knowledge it fears. Abraham Maslow, who wrote of the "need to know and fear of knowing," observed that "it is precisely the god-like in ourselves that we are ambivalent about, fascinated by and fearful of, motivated to and defensive against."[2]

Because the quest for knowledge and the fear of knowing are so central to human life, and to the human role in evolution, I would like to pause briefly over some fundamental points regarding information itself. First of all, evolution is learning. Evolution is often defined as gradual change, but this definition is slightly misleading. Learning processes are never merely gradual. If we look at the growth of a child, as it learns its way into adulthood, we see some steady and apparently gradual change—and also bewildering shifts, some of them abrupt and traumatic. The rate of learning sometimes changes, and at different stages of life the child concentrates on different things. It is forever learning and unlearning, putting its store of information together into new patterns. It learns some things unconsciously, and does not always know what it knows. It will go to great lengths to obtain some kinds of information, and to equally great lengths to avoid other kinds. It learns about learning, and learns how to learn.

The evolution of organic life on Earth—a learning process infinitely more complicated, more sinuous in its twists and turns and changes of form—has involved two different kinds of information with two different ways of passing that information along. The two kinds of information are genetic and symbolic.

The locus of genetic information—and the key to genetic evolution—is the DNA molecule, which has the marvelous ability to duplicate itself and thus to produce a new cell wherein is encoded the same information and abilities.

The other kind of information is in symbols and is passed along from generation to generation by means of speech and writing. Other species show rudimentary forms of symbolic communication, but the human capacity turned into something quite different from anything that previously existed on Earth, and the appearance of speech—an "event" that must have taken thousands of years—marks an evolutionary turning-point whose importance can scarcely be overestimated. It has been described by biologists as the appearance of a fundamentally new sort of evolution, marked by a new sort of heredity.[3] Symbols greatly increased the amount and kind of information that could be passed on from one generation to the next. Some call this system "cultural DNA" or the "sociogenetic transfer system." These are difficult terms—when it comes to describing itself, the symbolic system is not elegant—but still serve as useful indicators of something central to all our lives.

When the symbolic information system appeared, so did human life; the two are synonymous. The symbolic capacity brought about a transformation of both social interaction and inner experience for *Homo sapiens*. First, it permitted the creation of a new kind of sociocultural environment—an environment of words—which extended in time and space far beyond the boundaries of families and tribes. It gave wider reach to the individual mind, and new kinds of information which gradually expanded to include technology and taboo, history and myth, poetry and theology. Simultaneously, it expanded the inward range of experience. When culture is internalized, its language and visual images become parts of the individual consciousness. The process permits an enormous widening of the range of mental experience, but (since some of what we internalize are rules and demands) also constricts experience. This is undoubtedly part of the reason for our mixed feelings about the gift of intelligence. The symbolic capacity becomes an inhibitor of actions; it descends like a curtain between the animal nature of the organism and its doings in the world, separates stimulus from response and instinct from gratification. The capacity to reason and consider alternatives, the insistent presence of cultural values, shut us out from the garden of animal innocence. They bring a tremendous richness to life, widen the dimensions of consiousness, and also—as Freud and his followers remind us—cause suffering and inner conflict.

As speech (and later, writing) transformed human society and human consciousness, it also transformed the biosphere. This is an aspect of the evolutionary process that we have overlooked: The appearance of a new system of information transfer changed the conditions of survival for all life. As the late T. H. Waddington used to say, "evolution evolves." A world that contains a species capable of thinking and communicating in symbols is different from a world that does not, since speech infinitely multiplies the species' impacts upon its environment. Evolution itself begins to operate according to a new set of rules.

Because the appearance of speech took place over such a long stretch of centuries, its beginnings lost in the prehistoric past (history itself was one of its products) we do not readily grasp the cause-and-effect sequence. Yet it is there: When the primitive grunts and cries of our ancestors became speech, the change set in motion a sequence of events that would extinguish thousands of species of plant and animal life, create new life forms through artificial breeding and genetic engineering, change the shape of the land and the contents of the air and water, produce theories of evolution and endangered species laws, and scatter debris on the moon. The developments unfolded so slowly that for many thousands of years the "symbolic animal" (as philosopher Ernst Cassirer called it) was able to conceal the truth from itself—something it passionately desired to do.

Homo Intervenor and the Prometheus Complex

THE DEVELOPMENT of the human species was accompanied by an increasing capacity to intervene in the evolutionary fortunes of other species—directly and indirectly, deliberately and accidentally. *Homo sapiens* could as accurately be called *Homo intervenor*, the tireless modifier of environments and manipulator of plant and animal life.

Consider a few of the early adventures, such as the capture of fire. Fire must have been the most awesome force in the environment: the lightning bolt from the sky, the destroyer. First, we surmise, it was avoided and feared, then carefully approached for warmth, and eventually semi-domesticated. When brands from wild fires were used to start a campfire the element became a tool, useful for cooking food and frightening away animals. And then over time, through applications of effort and ingenuity that make the triumphs of modern science seem modest by comparison, somebody or many somebodies figured out how to start fires. All this adds up to a majestic human accomplishment, and it led to alterations of environments on a scale that would boggle the mind of Smokey the Bear—because, once people got the hang of fire-making, they used fire prodigiously: used it to burn away forests and increase the yield of edible grasses or berries, used it in hunting, used it in war, used it to create habitats for the species they hunted. The American Indians, romanticized by modern Americans as the great non-intervenors, burned happily from Tierra del Fuego to the Arctic Circle, and so did their counterparts in every other part of the world, with environmental effects that have only recently been discovered. Over the past few decades evidence has mounted that many ecosystems once considered "natural"—such as the African savannas—were enlarged (if not produced) by human intervention, with fire as a major tool. Fire also became an agricultural tool: Ancient Chinese records dating from about 8000 B.C. mention the practice of clearing new farmland by burning off the trees and underbrush and then flooding it—and the practice was probably millennia old by then.[4]

Every increase of human ability to insure food supplies affected other species and their environments. Domestication of animals probably began with the dog, and then proceeded to the use of decoys in hunting—a female deer, for example, to lure a buck or distract the attention of a herd. Decoy animals were bred in captivity, their captors evolving gradually from hunters to herdsmen. In other cases, herding may have been a progression from herd-following, using animals for their milk or fur; dogs probably assisted in these early domestications of other species. The domestication of animals became more sophisticated with selective breeding—a whole new order of intervention in which the evolution of some species began to be determined by human criteria rather than by the capacity of an individual animal to survive in its environment. Another consequence of advanced domestication was movement of species from their native habitats. Reindeer were herded in the same regions where they had run wild, but other animals found themselves in new environments: Wild goats and sheep, which had originally inhabited mountains and high hillsides, were herded on the plain; wild cattle were similarly moved far from the forests and savannas they had once occupied. A rock painting at Tassili in the central Sahara shows men with herds of oxen. The painting dates from the time when parts of the Sahara were grassland, and the herdsmen may have come from the Nile valley 1500 miles away.[5] Herding brought a new kind of relationship between human and animal—consider the imagery of the Twenty-Third Psalm—in which the human's role was to protect the herd against the dangers of a strange environment. And wherever animals moved into new green pastures, secondary effects resulted—from grazing, from the movement of diseases and pests and predators, from the accidental transportation of seeds and spore. We know what happened when the Spanish brought a few animals to California, and can surmise that similar changes resulted from the movement of domesticated animals across Asia, Africa and Europe in earlier times.

Human evolution led to similar changes in the evolution of plants: Even before people began planting seeds and tubers and cuttings to grow food, they were harvesting wild-growing plants such as wheat and barley, and getting good at it: Archaeologists have discovered flint-bladed sickles and grain-milling tools among the relics of hunter-gatherer tribes. As people moved into the stage of true agriculture, ecosystems changed: Land was cleared by burning or cutting forests and brush, animal habitats were destroyed, and plants were moved from place to place.

In the same way that ideas pass from one society to another in the process called cultural diffusion, the seeds of food plants moved slowly around the world. Rice, one of the most traveled of prehistoric food sources, was probably first grown in Southeast Asia, then spread through China and India and eventually to Africa and Europe. All of the world's major food crops were in use before the beginning of recorded history, and all of them come from a few natural homelands. The Russian botanist N. I. Vavilov found that all the plants we depend on for food originated on less than one quarter of the world's arable land, in the regions of genetic diversity now called Vavilov Centers—in such regions as the Mediterranean, the Near East, Afghanistan, Indo-Burma, Malaysia-Java, Guatemala-Mexico, the Peruvian Andes, and Ethiopia. The movement of domesticated food plants around the world inevitably brought a host of lesser interventions. Plants do not travel alone any more than animals do, and their movement to a new home always involved some remodeling of the property.

Several inventions—such as the plow—helped the course of agriculture along. The most important agricultural invention was the development of irrigation. Here and there, on a small scale, people had dug ditches and diverted small amounts of water, but in Egypt and Mesopotamia—and later in other places—they dug large canals, built levees, in effect created artificial rivers and streams. This was much more than an invention; it was a complex piece of human progress that involved new knowledge, increased control over the environment, and new political orders. One of the consequences of the development of speech is a vastly expanded ability to organize. People do not merely survive in different terrains and climates, but organize to do so. The organizational patterns of other social animals are mostly dependent on genetic information and vary only minutely over space and time. To survive under radically different conditions they have to progress through the slow and costly route of genetic evolution. Since they are limited in their capacity to adapt by reorganizing and altering their environments, they can adapt only by becoming different life forms.

The human species, in a burst of social/technological creativity a few thousand years before the time of Christ, invented new organizations—the irrigation system, the city—which were simultaneously new political systems and new ecosystems.

Irrigation required much thought and planning, some division of labor, tiers of leadership, and maintenance of the system over time. It produced irrigated land and improved food supplies and increased human populations— and also produced centralized governments, social stratification, and bureaucracy. Karl Wittfogel, the great scholar of the politics of irrigation, more or less equates the ancient "hydraulic civilizations" with Oriental despotism.[6]

THE CITY was another human invention, another artificial ecosystem, another kind of social order. The walled city is a fundamentally different thing from a village, just as a true hydraulic civilization is different from a place where a few farmers dig a ditch or two. It calls into being a new mode of organization—a government—and it vastly expands the ability of the people involved to transform their environment. For the first time, people could live out their lives in surroundings that were clearly human creations, and that provided an unprecedented degree of protection from enemies and predators, from the weather, and from fire—the latter a matter of increasing importance as papyrus and paper came into general use. All of the city's structures—walls, houses, roads, reservoirs, sewers, aqueducts—were barricades against the dangers and uncertainties of the natural environment. "Standing out in the vegetation-clad landscape," Lewis Mumford writes, "the city became an oasis of stone or clay."[7] Usually that vegetation-clad landscape was a domesticated one of plowed field and meadow, where food crops grew and herds of tame animals grazed. No ancient city—any more than any modern one—was sufficient unto itself. Its survival depended upon a steady supply of food, fiber, metal, and water. It thus altered the land upon which it stood and the rivers that flowed by or through it, and extended its impact to the surrounding terrain and—as cities became larger, their technologies more advanced, their aspirations more grandiose—to distant lands and even to other continents. The Romans denuded forest areas far from the mother city to provide fuel for their baths and centrally heated palaces and for their smelters and forges and kilns. The dining tables of the aristocracy were supplied with food from every corner of the empire.

The city-dwellers knew or cared little about such distant impacts; urban life was increasingly an existence amid words and symbols, human relationships and human artifacts. They worried less about the perils of nature, worried more about each other and about their powerful rulers. The institution of kingship—a new kind of concentration of authority—appears to have been an integral part of the new urban mode of organization. Just as the city was a giant step beyond the settlements that had preceded it, so was the sovereign king—with his ability to command and direct the efforts of his subjects to goals of his choosing—different from the tribal or village chieftain. The authority of early kings was so great that it was commonly justified as expressing the will of the gods. Some kings were priests and some persuaded their subjects (and themselves) that they were gods incarnate. Some societies, in a rough step toward constitutional governance, mitigated royal authority by the not altogether unreasonable device of giving the king unlimited power for a limited time and then killing him.[8]

Civilized life brought great advances in human knowledge and many benefits: material goods, food supplies, protection, new entertainments and conviviality, and the excitement and pride of being a part of such grandeur. It also brought regimentation, harsh laws, grinding work, tyranny, and warfare. The early city-state, like the modern nation-state, was an instrument of war. Some early civilizations were destroyed by their enemies; some by disease (plagues were one of the biological characteristics of urban life); some by natural disasters such as flood or drought; and some, like Babylon, by their own depredations on the environments that had sustained them. Civilized life was far from risk-free, then; it had its own kinds of catastrophes, and they were often on a heroic scale.

It is hard to imagine how life really felt for people in the early cities, but there is abundant evidence that, whatever the comforts, people commonly experienced a sense of loss and dreamed of times when things had been simpler. We think of the back-to-nature urge as a modern phenomenon, but the bards of Sumeria, at the very dawn of history, were already singing of a legendary past era when "there was no fear, nor terror," and "man had no rival." Stories of a lost golden age appear again and again in the unearthed lore of early civilizations and they tell us that the human species has always, in the corner of its collective mind where myths live, contemplated its forward progress with fear and dreamt of days gone by. It has become a common figure of speech in our time, referring to this or that benighted conservative, to say he has had to be dragged kicking and screaming into the twentieth century, but in fact the human species has had to be dragged kicking and screaming into every century. There is much pain in evolution, but only the human species experiences the pain of life in the symbolic dimension, in history—with the sense of being always at the edge, leaving the past behind, taking on new powers, setting in motion lines of action whose final outcomes cannot be predicted.

NOBODY expressed this feeling more eloquently than the Greeks. A striving people whose record of discovery and learning still astounds us, they had their own legends of a past golden age and must have felt deeply the fear of knowledge and progress. They produced powerful and vivid mythic images of it: Pandora's box, Prometheus the fire-bringer. The Prometheus myth is as much a part of Western culture as Genesis, and it deals with the same subject: the danger of acquiring knowledge. Prometheus stole fire from the gods, gave it to human beings to bring them out of their pre-human condition, and was sentenced to eternal punishment for it. In Aeschylus' dramatic retelling of the Promethean story—the version best-known in ancient Greece—the meaning of the act expands beyond the gift of fire and becomes the gift of knowledge itself. Prometheus' name means "Forethought" or "Forethinker." In the play, chained to the mountains where his fate is to have his liver endlessly devoured by a vulture, Prometheus speaks of his gift as a gift of knowledge and affirms the rightness of what he has done:

> I speak to you who know.
> Hear rather that all mortals suffered.
> Once they were fools. I gave them power to think.
> Through me they won their minds.[9]

[37]

Like Genesis, the Promethean myth expresses the fear that when knowledge is acquired somebody is going to get in trouble for it. Genesis, reflecting the Judeo-Christian taste for guilt, gets the whole human race in trouble— exiled for all time from Paradise. The Prometheus myth is a scapegoat story; it lets the hero suffer alone, Christ-like, taking on the burden of a crime against the gods while the human race is permitted to enjoy his gift. But we should not forget that Pandora is also part of the Greek story of creation (in fact she is the first woman, the counterpart of Eve) and that her box is full of troubles for the human race; everything except that one item at the very bottom, Hope, is an ailment of the body or the mind.

The moral of such myths, deep and persistent themes in the folklore of so many civilizations, is a warning against acquiring knowledge. The myths enact the drama of humanity's search for its proper role in the scheme of things; they show the human species emerging out of an animal-like condition but in the process trespassing upon forbidden territory and incurring divine wrath. They are cautionary tales, but we note that the societies that invented them did not follow their own advice: They went right ahead learning, discovering, inventing, endlessly re-creating their societies and their environments. The Athenians who sat in the amphitheatre and shuddered at the punishment of Prometheus were the same people who applauded their countrymen's achievements in science and philosophy.

This might seem contradictory, but it is a contradiction endemic to the species. We can frighten ourselves with stories about the consequences of acquiring knowledge, but we do not know how to stop our own learning nor do we know how to prevent others from searching for new knowledge. Organized religions and other power

[38]

structures have made impressive efforts in regard to the latter, but with little success. The lust for knowledge is as strong in its own way as the more primal drives—as we see in the story of Faust, another myth in the Promethean tradition. One of the richest of evolution's many ironies is that the human species appears to be powerfully driven by its genetic nature to seek and communicate symbolic information.

The Idea of Progress and the Idea of Evolution

THE EXPLOSION of creativity that was classical Greece brought forth new understanding about many subjects, including the organization of human societies. The Athenians established an admirable system of government, and also produced the first systematic studies of governance itself—in the works of Plato and Aristotle, a new and essentially hopeful political philosophy. The idea of the polis, as expressed in Greek philosophy, is as much an evolutionary leap as the invention of monarchy and the city-state had been. It is an immensely humanized vision, which equates the interests of the state with those of its citizens; the state's function is to complete the task genetic evolution had left unfinished and make human beings truly human: "For Man," wrote Aristotle, "when perfected, is the best of animals, but, when separate from law and justice, he is the worst of all."[10] The idea of the human species as a political animal was a profound insight into human nature. It recognized the need for more than mere biological growth and survival within the herd. It envisioned a wider context, the polis, within which the individual could realize his or her potential. It was an integral part of this vision that citizenship was a two-way proposition, that self-development involved contribution to the well-being of the larger organism of which the individual was a part. And, by the very act of studying different political systems, analyzing their good and bad aspects, Aristotle demonstrated that the form of the state was an artifact, a thing of human making whose principles could be discovered. His work grew out of the knowledge that the political animal is not only the citizen of the polis, but the creator of it.

Aristotle would never have been the kind of political philosopher he was if he had not also been a student of biology. He observed the behavior of other animals, noted their various social systems, and pondered the question of what it was that made human beings different from—as he put it—"bees and other gregarious animals." The difference was the polis, he concluded, and the root cause was the power of speech, which made the creation of the polis possible. He discovered what twentieth century political scientists would rediscover, which is that the state is a communications system. He put the matter in a richer framework of thought than modern political theorists do, uniting political and moral concepts with biological ones.

The Greek civilization of Aristotle's time was just primitive enough that it was still possible for one person to inquire into both governance and the non-human realm of plant and animal life. Even then there was a tendency to separate the two: Aristotle had no concept of an ecosystem, and he did not seriously address himself to the question of whether a polis, in occupying a portion of the Earth's territory, did not perhaps alter the terrain and have impacts on the non-human life forms that also occupied it. From Aristotle's time onward the two subjects—the political and the biological—took different paths.

Sometimes they bumped into one another in the dark: Political philosophers often talked about how natural environments affected human civilizations, but not much attention was paid to how civilizations affected natural environments.

Aristotle was occupied with the task of studying all observable living species. This was in itself a great step along the evolutionary road. People had always been fascinated students of other life forms, but Aristotle was surveying a wider territory—the entire known world—and was looking for ways that all living species might be identified and classified, perhaps hierarchically. He was trying to understand organic life on Earth in its totality, as some kind of system.

Aristotle's biological work laid the foundation for what Arthur Lovejoy called "one of the most grandiose enterprises of the human intellect"—the slowly-developed concept of a Great Chain of Being, a systematically ordered world with a perfect gradation from one life form to the next and a continuity linking them all: inert matter at the bottom, God at the top, and humankind among the upper middle classes.[11] This huge theory-building project continued for more than two thousand years and had its greatest flowering in the eighteenth century. Its basic belief was that God had created all beings and had assigned them to their various places; within this belief system there was room for endless disputation of the sort at which medieval intellectuals excelled—debating the fine points of the Maker's intent, and laboring over the nuances of whether He had or had not created everything He was capable of creating, forged every conceivable link in the Great Chain. As science progressed, it became the work of God-fearing naturalists to get this concept down into precise terms, which meant classifying every living thing into its appropriate position in the hierarchy.

The prevailing view was that the hierarchy was fixed for all time, that the creation of Adam and Eve had been the final and consummate act which completed the picture and finished the task. The Abbe Pluché expressed this position well in the early eighteenth century when, having reviewed the thinking on the subject, he wrote: "Nothing more, therefore, will be produced in all the ages to follow. All the philosophers have deliberated and come to agreement upon this point. Consult the evidence of experience; elements always the same, species that never vary, seeds and germs prepared in advance for the perpetuation of everything . . . so that one can say, Nothing new under the sun, no new production, no species which has not been since the beginning." [12]

Nothing new added and nothing old lost: It was essential to this view of things that the chain be complete, and it was therefore unthinkable that any species might become extinct. "One step broken," wrote Alexander Pope, "the great scale's destroyed." [13]

The Great Chain of Being was the reigning view in theology and the natural sciences and it influenced the way people thought about the political order. The hierarchical view of plant and animal life could easily apply to the social classes. If every fish and flower had its place in the Creation—an unchanging place—then did it not follow that every person had his or her place, and that the essence of civic duty was to stay there? It is hard for Americans, reared in the land of Horatio Alger, to remember that there were social orders in which "keeping one's station" was not only good citizenship but true Christianity. This world-view also provided an answer of sorts to the troublesome question of why life in the existing political orders was so obviously fraught with injustice, misery, dissatisfaction and violent death. The answer was that the human species, occupying as it did an intermediate position in the chain, somewhere between the beasts and the angels, was not entitled to anything better. The eighteenth-century philosopher Soame Jenyns noted that there were "numberless imperfections inherent in all human governments . . . imputable only to the inferiority of man's station in the universe, which necessarily exposes him to natural and moral evils, and must, for the same reason, to political and religious . . . those grievous burdens of tyranny and oppression, of violence and corruption, of war and desolation, under which all nations have ever groaned on account of government."[14]

The Great Chain philosophy even managed to explain why God had created predatory animals. It was accepted by everyone that all nonhuman life forms had been created to serve humanity (a proposition that Lovejoy testily dismissed as "one of the most curious monuments of human imbecility") but this did not quite satisfactorily account for the existence of animals that preyed on domestic animals and, sometimes, on people. It was a tough theological question. The answer that the famous theologian François Fénelon gave, and which gained wide acceptance, was that the situation merely reflected another shortcoming of government: "If all countries were peopled and made subject to law and order as they should be, there would be no animals that would attack men."[15]

This view of the world did not incline greatly toward ideas of political and social improvement, and scholars have argued over whether there was, prior to modern times, any concept of human progress at all. The consensus used to be that there was not, or at any rate that such ideas were, in most civilizations, overshadowed by views of history as a fall away from a golden age, or as a cyclical recurrence like the seasons. More recently, sociologist/historian Robert Nisbet argued strongly that an idea of progress—of advancement through time out of barbarism toward a more desirable future—has been a persistent theme of human thought all through recorded history. He conceded, however, that this idea of progress has not been mere booster optimism, but a troubled and ambivalent view of cultural evolution: "There have been in the past, there are now, there always will be, no doubt, those who believe that . . . achievement of spiritual bliss and moral perfection demands, as its condition, not achievement or increase of knowledge—of world and man—but repudiation of such knowledge . . . . There hasn't been an age . . . in Western history in which some variant of this view of the inverse relation between happiness and knowledge hasn't had currency."[16]

Somehow people were able to maintain, over a period of thousands of years, a vision of a world in which all things subhuman remained precisely as they had been created—while the human race changed and developed, added to its store of knowledge, and (although there were serious doubts about this part) generally improved the quality of its existence. What is even more remarkable is that talk of human progress frequently dwelled on the increased capacity to make use of animals, convert wild land to agriculture, and otherwise master nature—without seriously considering that, by doing so, people were becoming active co-participants in the Creation.

Once in a while, there were stirrings of thought toward the belief that the Great Chain of Being might not be

[44]

static and perfect, that there might be some principle of progress—of evolution—applicable to the entire cosmos. The German philosopher Gottfried von Leibnitz, writing at the beginning of the eighteenth century, was one of the first to talk of such a principle. He believed that, "To realize in its completeness the universal beauty and perfection of the works of God, we must recognize a certain perpetual and very free progress of the whole universe, such that it is always going forward to greater improvement."[17]

By the late eighteenth century the idea of evolution was widely known, if not widely accepted. Although it had been expounded by thinkers as eminent as Leibnitz and Diderot, the idea that some sort of progress took place in the world of nature, that the Creation was still happening, was not yet quite respectable. One of its most enthusiastic advocates was the English physician Erasmus Darwin, a man who was well-known in his own time although today his memory has been overshadowed by that of his famous grandson Charles. Erasmus Darwin was not exactly the model of a modern scientist: He went in for wild speculations and florid writing, much of it in verse. Samuel Taylor Coleridge, who was impressed by neither the doctor's ideas nor his literary style, coined the word "Darwinizing" as a general label for what we would today call flaky thinking. Nevertheless, Dr. Darwin's books—*Zoonomia* and *Phytologia* and *The Botanic Garden*—were widely read, and introduced many people to the idea that the world of nature was a world of change. So did the French biologist Jean Baptiste Lamarck, whose work appeared later. (Lamarck's major book was published in the year of Charles Darwin's birth, 1809.) Lamarck theorized that the organs of animals changed according to how they were used or unused, and that these "acquired characteristics" were passed on to subsequent generations. He was one of several scientists, in England and on the continent, who were choosing up sides on the evolution issue: By 1830, about thirty years before Charles Darwin first made public his theory of natural selection, there was already a running battle between evolutionists and their opponents, who called themselves "immutabilists."

We are talking about a seedbed time: the period of a hundred and fifty years from 1750—the year the young French intellectual Turgot delivered his memorable lecture entitled "A Philosophical Review of the Successive Advances of the Human Mind," the first manifesto of the modern religion of progress—to the end of the nineteenth century. This was a period that can rightly be regarded as the beginning of the modern era. Science was on the march, religion was retreating into its compartment, and political upheavals were shaking the world. Western civilization was infatuated with the idea of progress, but opposition and reservations were surfacing in many forms. Clerics railed from their pulpits against placing human science above holy writ, and conservative thinkers such as Burke counseled great care in swallowing such heady phrases of the time as "the rights of man."

Pause a moment over Edmund Burke, M. P.: His writings are an important marker along the road of human evolution, because he was the first political thinker to develop what might be called a theory of conservatism. There had been plenty of conservative philosophers, sturdy defenders of the Divine Right of Kings and other bedrock principles of Christian monarchy—but nobody had tried to work out rules about political change itself. Burke, as a young man, championed the American revolution on the grounds that the American character and historical experience formed a sound basis for self-government. Later, when the French revolution began and many English took it to be essentially the same kind of phenomenon, Burke dissented. He had almost nothing good to say about the French revolution, which he saw as an unsound attempt to gallop from monarchy to democracy mounted on ideas instead of experience. He did not think highly of Rousseau and Voltaire, and spoke of French revolutionary theorizing as "the polluted nonsense of their most licentious and giddy coffeehouses." Burke was merely a politician of his time, busy in Parliament and party affairs, speaking out on the issues as they arose—but he was involved in an evolutionary enterprise no less momentous than the capture of fire. He was trying to make sense out of political progress, searching for rules about when and how it should proceed, and when and how it should be restrained.

There was much ferment about political progress, much ferment about progress in the realm of nature—and even, here and there, a few scattered suggestions that there might be some connection between the two. The most important link—the first real biopolitical issue to arise in modern times—was the question of what might be the result of human population growth. This subject came up frequently in the eighteenth and nineteenth centuries. It is an especially interesting line of inquiry to follow, because it leads us straight to Charles Darwin and to one of the greatest upheavals in the history of human thought.

Consider the Marquis de Condorcet, one of history's tragic and ironic figures: A nobleman, he was a passionate defender of the French revolution; though a revolutionist he got in trouble with the Jacobins and died, probably by his own hand, in prison, a few jumps ahead of the guillotine. Condorcet was certain that all science was forward motion toward human betterment, but he did have one nagging concern: He wondered if, as the human condition became ever more perfect and prosperous, there might not come a time "when the increase in the number of man (surpasses) that of their means," resulting in a "decrease in prosperity and in population," and perhaps "at least a sort of oscillation between the good and the bad . . . a constant source of almost periodical calamities?"[18]

Another utopian believer in progress, William Godwin in England, also gave some thought to whether overpopulation might be an obstacle to human progress. Neither Condorcet or Godwin really proved that this would be an insurmountable problem, but their writings inspired the reverend Thomas Malthus to compose his *Essay on Population*, which he described as "remarks on the speculations of Mr. Godwin, M. Condorcet, and other writers." Malthus here outlined his famous theory of geometrical population growth and arithmetical increase in food supply—and warned of a future very different from the perfected political society that the progressives expected. Malthus did not think the population problem necessarily ruled out all progress, and he corresponded amiably with Godwin on this subject after his essay was published—but he had brought into the dialogue a new issue, powerfully stated (overstated, in fact) and his theory has had a tremendous impact on human thinking. It was another one of those things that people were not at all sure they wanted to hear about, and much energy has been expended in the effort to prove that Malthus was completely off the page.

So, even in the booming decades when progress was virtually a religion, there were certain misgivings: hints of larger issues, suggestions that the human race had yet much to learn about its learning. William Godwin's daughter, Mary Shelley, contributed to that dialogue in her own way when she wrote her novel *Frankenstein, or, The Modern Prometheus*—the most famous modern fable of knowledge gone berserk, of power over nature exerted with tragic consequences. Dr. Frankenstein became the model for all the mad scientists who have rampaged through the motion pictures, ever disregarding the advice that There Are Some Things Not Meant for Man to Know. The standard modern horror movie is our myth of progress gone wrong, a replay of Genesis and Prometheus.

The appearance of the population issue was a harbinger, a prelude to larger evolutionary questions yet to be confronted. It was, of course, an evolutionary question: Human skills at survival had progressed to the point at which it became necessary to ask whether the species might not increase in numbers beyond the carrying capacity of the planet. The question was, from the very beginning, political, but the extent to which the human species was becoming capable of making decisions about the course of evolution, was not grasped by any of the participants in the population debate. Malthus does not seem to have been aware of any human impacts upon the Earth other than the desirable ones of bringing land under cultivation so it could produce food. One of the few forerunners of Darwin who did see that the human species had become a force in evolution was a French naturalist, Count Georges de Buffon; Buffon (Lamarck's mentor and patron) studied the cumulative effects of breeding plants and animals and modifying environments, and even discovered instances where human intervention, as in the clearing of forests, had resulted in climatic change. In his essay "Epochs of

Nature," he divided the Earth's history into seven periods, the last designated as the time "when the power of man assisted the works of nature."[19] Buffon was, as they say, ahead of his time.

So the culture into which Charles Darwin introduced his discoveries about the mechanism of species evolution was one that had already moved away from the static concept of the Great Chain of Being, and was getting ready to take the next step, into a progressive concept, a theory of evolution. Many people, in fact, had already taken the step. Henry Adams, an astute observer of the times, wrote that he felt, "like nine men in ten, an instinctive belief in Evolution. . . ." But there was no comparable readiness to take the step beyond that, the one Buffon had taken, and perceive that the human species was an active agent in evolution.

Even the relatively modest step that Darwin did take, in providing a documented and plausible explanation of how evolution worked, had what Adams called a "convulsing" effect on society. It took its toll on Darwin himself: He fell ill soon after his return from the voyage of the *Beagle*, and was an invalid for the remaining forty years of his life. The cause of the illness has never been explained; some think it was the result of a bite from an exotic insect, others believe it was psychosomatic. He started work on what became *The Origin of Species* in 1837, had completed a huge manuscript that he called an "essay" seven years later, and waited another fourteen years before deciding to publish it. He would not have done so even then had not another naturalist, Alfred Wallace, arrived independently at the same theory.

Darwin and Wallace were both naturalists who had formed their conclusions through direct observation, and both had been influenced by Malthus. Until he read Malthus' essay, Darwin had assumed that a species produced only enough offspring to maintain its position in nature.[20] The concept of excessive reproduction became a basic part of the theory of natural selection. In his introduction to *The Origin of Species*, Darwin spoke of "the Struggle for Existence amongst all organic beings throughout the world, which inevitably follows from the high geometrical ratio of their increase . . .," and called his theory of natural selection "the doctrine of Malthus, applied to the whole animal and vegetable kingdoms." His thesis was that, more individuals being born than can survive, those with any genetic characteristics that improved their chances would have been "naturally selected."[21]

The world of evolving nature that Darwin unveiled had a curiously robot-like character. There was no active consciousness in evolution beyond the survival instinct, and no symbolic information that played any part in the process. Darwin's accomplishment was remarkably similar to that of Isaac Newton: Newton had given the world an image of a mechanistic cosmos, operating according to laws that were discoverable by human consciousness but that had no discoverable intentionality in them. Darwin, like Newton, professed to see the hand of a Creator behind his vast machinery, but it proved to be no trouble at all for scientific Darwinists—no more than it had been for scientific Newtonians—to let the clockmaker fade away and deal only with the clock.

Although Darwin contributed but a piece of the evolutionary jigsaw puzzle it was the piece that made the difference, and he became the center of a huge controversy. Benjamin Disraeli, with a politician's flair for reducing all things to factional conflict, described the issue to a gathering of English clergymen as a dispute between those who saw the human species as ape and those who saw it as angel; he declared himself to be on the side of the angels. The controversy was not as cleanly divided along the religion-v.-science line as is commonly believed, however. Many members of the clergy accepted the principle of natural selection and revised their ideas about nature's workings accordingly. The custom of viewing the Bible as something other than a literal history was already well-established. Yet a powerful opposition movement did emerge, and its most prominent spokesman was the Bishop of Oxford, Samuel Wilberforce. It was the venerable Wilberforce who coined the most famous of all anti-Darwinian epigrams when he asked Darwin's colleague T. H. Huxley whether it was through his grandfather or his grandmother that he claimed descent from a monkey. (Huxley, who replied that he would rather be descended from an ape than from Bishop Wilberforce, is generally credited as the winner of the exchange.)

What people found most objectionable in Darwin's theory were ideas that seemed to diminish the stature of the human species: first, the implicit assertion that all the other species of plant and animal life had *not* been created specifically to be of service to people, but were instead shaped according to the mechanistic and quite impersonal laws of the evolutionary process; second, the idea that the human species was a part of the same process and probably descended from a non-human species. "Our unsuspected cousinship with the mushrooms," Bishop Wilberforce called it on one occasion. This, too, was not explicit in *The Origin of Species*; Darwin only suggested cautiously that "much light will be thrown on the origin of man and his history" as a result of future research and did not actually elaborate on the human-ape connection until many years later, in *Descent of Man*. He didn't have to: The society into which he introduced his ideas was already familiar with the general outlines of the argument, and most people already knew where they stood.

There is something amazingly contradictory about the way the Darwinian revolution actually took place. Gertrude Himmelfarb, its most perceptive historian, notes this and adds: "The anomaly increases as time goes on, as his predecessors seem to multiply in number, as the philosophical presuppositions of the theory are pushed farther back in time, as critics find more and more flaws in the theory and the passage of time brings its vindication no nearer—and as, in spite of all this, history persists in dividing itself into a pre-Darwin and a post-Darwin epoch."[22]

The anomaly has to do with the curious character of human knowing, with the way in which the human mind simultaneously pursues new comprehension and shrinks from its discoveries. Clearly, informed people already knew about evolution, and knew whether they liked the idea or not. Samuel Butler said: "Buffon planted, Erasmus Darwin and Lamarck watered, but it was Mr. Darwin who said, 'That fruit is ripe,' and shook it into his lap."[23] As Himmelfarb puts it, what people experienced on reading *The Origin of Species* "was not the shock of discovery but rather the shock of recognition."[24]

Scarcely less amazing is what they did *not* recognize, the part of Buffon's plant that did not bear fruit in the nineteenth century, the idea that was even simpler than natural selection—which was that the human species had discovered evolution and, by discovering it, changed it irrevocably. Darwin does not appear to have perceived

[53]

this himself. He described a mechanism of evolution without ever suggesting that a mechanism which figures out its own principles of operation is not a mechanism at all, but something far more intelligent and far more mysterious. His opponents clearly did not see this: When they protested that the theory of evolution was a denigration of the human species, they failed to consider that a species which can discover the principles of evolution—in a mere few thousand years from the beginning of its recorded history—is a remarkable beast indeed, and as much angel as ape. T.H. Huxley's grandson Julian caught the essence of this other discovery much later, when, in his introduction to a 1958 edition of *The Origin of Species* he said that, "in the light of the science of evolutionary biology which Darwin founded, man is seen not just as a part of nature, but as a very peculiar and indeed unique part. In his person the evolutionary process has become conscious of itself."[25]

Huxley's observation puts evolution in what we would today call a holistic or systemic frame of reference. Instead of perpetuating the schism between nature and humanity, between genetic information and symbolic information, between the thing known and the knower, it suggests a more richly unified view of a biosphere that changes as learning takes place within it. It is a world-view of a kind that Darwin did not possess.

Darwin and his society saw the world much as they saw England itself: a green and pleasant place, wherein some lands were cultivated and some not, some species domesticated and some not. Nearly everyone, regardless of what he or she believed about evolution, agreed that there was a distinct line to be drawn between the two, a place where the field ended and the forest began. Darwin did not disturb that consensus. He himself saw a clear distinction between the rules that applied in the evolution of domestic life forms—a subject about which he wrote a two-volume study—and the rules that applied in nature. In the former, human volition prevailed; in the latter, in nature, the rule was survival of the fittest, according to which the only thing that determined a species' success or failure was its ability to adapt to its environment. The idea that humans intervened in other ways—by modifying "natural" environments—was foreign to Darwin. There is a passage in *The Origin of Species* in which he compared the vegetation of a heath in Staffordshire to that in a similar area that had been enclosed and planted with Scotch fir. Darwin referred to the heath as having "never been touched by the hand of man," although it is quite likely that the heath had been a forest itself before it was denuded by woodcutters; much of England was so thoroughly logged over by the thirteenth century that trees were imported from the Baltic area, forerunners to the reforestation from Scotland that Darwin observed.[26]

In general people believed that human intervention was limited and benign. Herbert Spencer, who was highly influential in Darwin's time, made this a central part of the political culture of the time. Spencer was both a political theorist and a student of biology, and his thinking in both areas reflected the cult of progress at its cheerfully blinkered best. In politics he was one of the great spokesmen for a point of view that we would today call conservative, although in its own time it went by the name of liberalism: the philosophy of laissez-faire, of government as the enemy of the individual, of freedom in the economic realm as the producer of well-being for all. Spencer defended all freedoms, including freedom "to use the land," and stood in the line of descent from the early apostles of progress such as Turgot; progress, as he put it in his celebrated *Social Statics*, "is not an accident, but a necessity." Spencer equated progress in human society with evolutionary progress in the rest of the world, and in *The Principles of Biology* he described an inevitable forward march of civilization that would culminate in an increase of human population until it would reach its equilibrium, with the whole world cultivated like a garden.[27]

Spencer believed he had refuted Malthus; he saw no problem in human population growth, and he had no concept of the Lilliput effect. He did not know that human activity had produced as many deserts as it had gardens, and he did not suspect—even in an England where the factories' smoke already filled the air—that the free commercial activity he advocated might have destructive effects on life. He told the industrialists that it was perfectly fine for them to go ahead and do what they were doing and he was, not surprisingly, a great success in his time. His influence was so great in the industrializing United States that Justice Oliver Wendell Holmes found it necesary to remind his brethren on the Supreme Court, in his famous dissenting opinion in the case of *Lochner v. New York*, that *Social Statics* had not been enacted into constitutional law.

Spencer's work laid the foundations for the political ideology called Social Darwinism. Its central idea was "survival of the fittest" (a phrase coined by Spencer, not Darwin, although Darwin later borrowed it) which became a rationale for unfettered capitalism, imperialism, and racism. Wherever there was an individual with greater power or wealth than others, or a nation or a race gaining ascendancy over another, the Social Darwinists took it to be the healthy working-out of the laws of nature to the eventual betterment of society as a whole. Prof. William Graham Sumner of Yale, one of the great boosters of Social Darwinism in the United States, said that millionaires were "a product of natural selection, acting on the whole body of men. . . . they may fairly be regarded as the naturally selected agents of society for certain work. They get high wages and live in luxury, but the bargain is a good one for society."[28]

The Social Darwinists prided themselves on the tough-mindedness of their world-view, and generally opposed actions by government that would interfere with the necessary "weeding out" of unfit individuals. Spencer had at least pretended to be a student of biology, but most Social Darwinists had little use for the life sciences except as a convenient resource bank from which could be drawn unexamined political doctrines useful to reinforce a strongly individualistic view of life in the modern world.

Despite Social Darwinism's overlay of progressivism in its reverence for technology and enterprise, it was essentially a regressive doctrine that tried to reduce human activity to the same set of rules which—so went the general belief of the time—applied in the realm of nature. It made the same mistake that Darwin had made: Darwin had underestimated the extent to which human activity shaped the "natural" environment, and the Social Darwinists underestimated the extent to which human activity shaped the social environment. They wanted to believe that free-market capitalism was the "natural" order of things; they looked away from all the evidence that it was in fact an exquisitely complex human creation, built with a vast body of theory, nourished by myth and theology (the famed Protestant Ethic) and maintained by the power of governments. Having systematically repressed the knowledge that social environments are human creations, Social Darwinists were generally hostile toward all reformist or utopian urges toward creating new social environments.

Social Darwinism was a child of confusion, a symptom of one of the most profound dislocations the human species has ever experienced: the transition from the sublime orderliness of the Great Chain of Being to the fearful uncertainties of a world in evolution. It was a transition in which the human species literally lost its place, for lack of a new vision of humanity as discoverer of evolution and intervenor in its processes. The Social Darwinist worldview was enthusiastic about the human ability to domesticate animals and cultivate land, but had nothing to say about other kinds of intervention. This was a remarkable oversight, since the British empire—at its very peak in Darwin's time—was one of the greatest machines for ecosystem-alteration ever created. It had imposed huge plantations of cash crops—rubber, tea, opium, tobacco—upon the ecosystems of distant regions of the world; its ships crossed all the oceans, moving plants and animals and people from one place to another; it had repopulated much of North America, Australia and Africa with its white-skinned citizens. It also, almost casually, sponsored scientific study of nature around the world, collection and categorization of data and samples of flora and fauna. In such work aboard one of Her Majesty's ships, the *Beagle*, Darwin made the observations that were the basis of *The Origin of Species*. The theory itself was a by-product of empire.

Human ability to intervene in nature was increasing majestically during the time when people were choosing up sides between the apes and the angels. New machines were processing food and fiber, human numbers were increasing, and so was human mobility. At the same time that Darwinian ideas were being fashioned into a simplistic political doctrine based on the survival of the fittest as the rule of life in society, developments in science and technology were making the same principle obsolete in the world of nature—making nature ever less "natural" and more accessible to human manipulation.

A few years after the publication of *The Origin of Species*, the modern science of genetics was born. Darwin had provided the theoretical framework; the Austrian monk Gregor Mendel performed the first systematic experimentation. Mendel had read Darwin; Darwin, unfortunately, never knew of Mendel's discoveries. Mendel worked with peas—peas of different shapes and sizes, round peas and wrinkled ones, yellow peas and green peas. In the process he went farther than Darwin had traveled, into the laws of inheritance: He discovered dominant and recessive traits. He read the results of his experimentation to the natural history society in the town of Brunn in 1866, and there is no record that anybody who was present at that event recognized it as a major forward step in human knowledge, evolution becoming conscious of another part of itself. The paper was forgotten, then rediscovered in 1900—rediscovered independently by three different researchers in three different countries. Rapid strides were being made in the technology of microscopy, and Mendel provided the theoretical framework that gave it meaning. The terminology of the infant science soon became more precise: Where a few years earlier students of inheritance had spoken of "bits" and "gemmules," they now spoke of "chromosomes" and "genes". The British zoologist William Bateson named the new science "genetics". Many of the geneticists followed Mendel's lead in experimentation, and soon their laboratories teemed with animal and plant life. A student of Bateson's, T. H. Morgan, discovered the usefulness of the *Drosophila* fruit fly, an ancient pest which now took on a certain charm by virtue of its ability to produce a new generation every two or three weeks. One scientist places Drosophila among "man's most important domesticates," right up there with the dog and the horse, because of its services in behalf of genetic science.[29]

Genetics had been an art long before it became a science, and Europe was already populated with many varieties of life, from roses to racehorses, that were products of generations of careful human intervention and not survivors in the hardball game of natural selection. It did not take long for the new discoveries of the post-Mendelians to find application on the farms and in the gardens. Genetic science revolutionized plant and animal breeding and also gave tremendous assistance to fledgling sciences such as immunology—and thus, indirectly, to improvements in disease control and to further increases in human population. An ironic development, since the issue of overpopulation was what had triggered the series of intellectual events that produced genetics.

While the practical effects of genetics rippled outward into the world, the science itself progressed with amazing speed. By the 1930s the charge was being led by the molecular biologists, students of the gene's chemistry; a couple of decades later, amid a flurry of ambition, greed, hard feelings, and Nobel prizes, the DNA molecule yielded up the secret of its structure. With that discovery, the door to the science and technology of genetic engineering swung open and the rules of evolution changed again.

In this remarkable series of developments, the human species managed to go through profound changes in its ability to intervene, without correspondingly revising its ideas about what was natural and what was not. The true extent of human alteration of the "natural" world was simply not a part of the public dialogue. I can think of three possible explanations for this. One (the hardest to justify, as we will see in a later chapter) is that adequate information was not available, that people simply did not know that their ancestors had stripped forests, drained marshes, changed the course of rivers, and carried plant and animal life here and there about the world, intervening in the workings of every ecosystem into which human life had penetrated. The second possible interpretation, which we might call the economic one, was that people did not want to be bothered with anything that got in the way of their doing what they wanted to do—exploit resources and prosper—and deliberately ignored any evidence tending to contradict the Spencerian creed that progress, prosperity, and evolutionary improvement were all of a piece. The third possibility, the one Genesis and the Greek myths suggest, is that people could not bear the crushing psychological burden of having taken on such power and responsibility.

Whatever the reasons, the avoidance pattern prevailed—and prevails still. Its days are numbered, however; our biological impact upon the world is rapidly taking on new dimensions, and presenting itself in ways that we cannot long ignore. We are about to discover that we have truly left the garden.

[3]

Shooting the
Genetic Rapids

THE ADVENT of environmentalism was one of the major
political events of the twentieth century. It was a messenger,
although at first none of us knew precisely what the message
was. People on the Right thought environmentalism was
a new assault on free enterprise. People on the Left thought
it was a plaything of white liberal elites. Many environmentalists thought it was a return to nature. Many jour-
nalists, accustomed to viewing American politics as a series
of fads, thought this was yet another one and wondered
when it would go away.

It has not gone away but has abided and grown; it has
institutionalized itself in political parties and international
organizations and legal structures at every level of government. We are beginning to recognize that environmentalism is not merely another special cause but a basic
dimension of governance, one that we had managed for
a long time to overlook but can overlook no longer. The
message of environmentalism is simply that the human

species has reached the point of being responsible for the basic infrastructure of its organic existence. The impacts of our numbers and technology are now such that the results of careless actions can no longer be absorbed invisibly by the air and water or passed along carelessly to future generations. Environmentalism is inseparably connected to that other modern phenomenon that is sometimes called the Information Revolution—the increase in the volume of data and ability to handle it that has resulted from various latter-day developments of the Industrial Revolution. For a long time there was no environmental movement because there was not very much information about environmental impacts. The impacts have been increasing in modern times, and information about the impacts has been increasing also. The first environmental concerns triggered a boom in scientific analysis and data-collection—which is one of the reasons environmental concern did not ebb away, as some thought it might, after a few safeguards were put in place. By providing support for environmental information-gathering, governments insure that the public continues to get the message—to be regularly reminded that modern life involves environmental dangers and environmental responsibility.

While we struggle with that message—it is another one of those things we would as soon not know—a second messenger comes down the path. This time the message is not only about the environment but about the totality of life on the planet, and about evolution. It has to do with a process of genetic change now taking place in the world, a process which was set in motion by human action and whose future course will be determined by other human actions.

[63]

In order to get a clear picture of the genetic rapids through which the world is now traveling, let us first take a look at what we know of the evolutionary record: It shows species appearing, existing with or without variations over long periods of time, and in some cases becoming extinct when individual members can no longer survive and breed in their environments. While there is much debate about the timing and specific mechanisms of this process, any scientist would agree that it unfolded very slowly. The rate of extinction of species, even at a time of rapid change such as the end of the Cretaceous period when the dinosaurs disappeared—the time now known as the "Great Extinction"—was probably around one per thousand years. Many species have lasted unchanged for millions of years, and the appearance of new species has been an equally leisurely process. The "rapid" evolution of mammals after the age of dinosaurs, for example, produced whales from their terrestial mammalian ancestors in something less than twelve million years. The modern punctuationalists, the biological speedsters who believe that new species evolve more quickly than Darwin thought, support their theory with such evidence as the appearance of new species of cichlid fish in a small lake in Uganda in something less than four thousand years from the time the lake became a separate body of water.[1] This is referred to as a "brief instant" in geological and evolutionary time—which it is, but it is also an instant that encompasses most of human history.

In contrast to this majestic scale of time let us consider the fact that the Earth is now undergoing a period of genetic change more rapid and more extensive than any known to the paleobiologists—measurable within decades, accelerating, and revealed by evidence far less speculative than any upon which we base our understanding of how the dinosaurs went and the whales came.

There are four identifiable aspects of this new process of rapid genetic change: The first is a rising rate of extinction of species. The second is a loss of genetic variation within some species: those upon which the major portion of the human race depends for food. The third is a quantum leap in human ability to intervene in evolutionary processes: genetic technology. The fourth is increasing transfer of life forms between ecosystems and continents. These four phenomena are separable as matters for study and discussion, but as we will see they interconnect in many ways. They relate to one another in the same way that economic indicators relate to one another: They are all messages about the same reality. That reality is a world which is changing biologically more rapidly than ever before—a world in which these changes are guided and influenced by many different fragmented public policies, and in which no government anywhere has a coherent general policy or even a clear knowledge of what it is doing. Let us look at each of these four aspects in turn. First, species loss:

The Second Great Extinction

PALEOBIOLOGISTS, reading the story inscribed by fossils in the Earth's crust, believe that about 65 million years ago a major evolutionary event took place. Over a period of some thousands of years, many species became extinct— apparently as a result of change in the earth's atmosphere. The climatic change may have been caused by geological forces such as continental drift; it may have been caused (as some scientists believe) by the collision of one or more asteroids with the Earth.

We noted that the rate of extinction during that cataclysm—whatever its cause—was about one species per thousand years. After the Great Extinction the rate apparently dropped, and has only begun to rise again in the very recent evolutionary past. We are now well into the second Great Extinction. By the year 1600 A.D., when the human species became capable of over-hunting animals and extensively disrupting environments, the rate of extinction began to rise rapidly, to about one species every four years. In the twentieth century it has risen with what looks like an exponential rate of change. Norman Myers estimates that one million species will be eliminated in the final quarter of this century—that the world is currently losing about one species per day and will very soon be losing one per hour.[2]

One reason the numbers are so high is that human populations have increased in regions where there is a great diversity of life forms. In terms of sheer numbers of species, this has been especially serious in tropical forests, which contain hundreds of thousands of as-yet-unclassified species of plants and insects, and which are being rapidly depleted by roadbuilding and forest clearing. Other causes of species extinction are overexploitation (of whales, for example); effects of industrial and agricultural chemicals—especially spraying of pesticides and herbicides; poaching and global trade in rare species; predator control (direct attacks against animals such as wolves which are perceived as being dangerous to domestic animals); urbanization and conversion of habitat to agricultural use (such as cattle grazing land); desertification from overgrazing or water diversion or firewood collection; land conversions such as flooding or draining; and expanding recreational uses, especially with off-road vehicles.[3]

The changes are happening most spectacularly in the tropical forests, but the phenomenon is not confined to any part of the world or to any specific class of life. Extinction is touching the entire world and threatening species of all kinds—from simple organisms to advanced primates such as humanity's closest relative, the chimpanzee. The estimates I have quoted above are disputed by some scientists who think they are too high and by others who think they are too low. They are definitely estimates and should not be treated as "hard data," but the basic process is well-documented. The rate of extinction is rising; it is an unprecedented and global phenomenon; and it is caused by human action.

This issue remains something of a sleeper, although many scientists place it near the top of the list of things the world should be taking seriously. Edward Wilson writes:

What event likely to happen during the next few years will our descendants most regret? Everyone agrees, defense ministers and environmentalists alike, that the worst thing possible is global nuclear war. If it occurs the entire human species is endangered; life as normal human beings wish to live it would come to an end. With that terrible truism acknowledged, it must be added that if no country pulls the trigger the worst thing that will *probably* happen—in fact is already well underway—is not energy depletion, economic collapse, conventional war, or even the expansion of totalitarian governments. As tragic as these catastrophes would be for us, they can be repaired within a few generations.

The one process now going on that will take millions of years to correct is the loss of genetic and species diversity by the destruction of natural habitats. This is the folly our descendants are least likely to forgive us.[4]

There have been various institutional responses to the rising rate of extinction—endangered species legislation, state and local habitat preserves, efforts by private organizations such as the Nature Conservancy, international conferences—but this ponderous mobilization is not proceeding with any speed comparable to that of the process it seeks to reverse. The issue's visibility is low, its constituency small. Even among environmentalists there is not much clarity of purpose. Environmental activists coalesce to protect this or that endangered species (usually the more attractive or interesting ones) but are less likely to unite behind obscure tropical insects—one can hardly expect anybody to take a stand for the preservation of something that hasn't even been discovered yet—or behind the somewhat amorphous problem of extinction itself.

Genetic Erosion

WHILE THE number of species and subspecies surviving in the wild declines—massively altering the character of the biosphere—a corresponding process of change is taking place among the domesticated life forms that are our major sources of food and fiber. Here the issue is not so much the extinction of species as the shrinking of genetic diversity within species.

If somebody were to write a science-fiction story about a planet in which the dominant species had begun to direct the evolutionary fortunes of other life forms, the writer might describe a remote site where the genetic resources of the planet were kept and protected against catastrophe—a gene storage center, a sort of biological Fort Knox. Its most precious treasures would be the seeds of the food plants that sustained the lives of members of the dominant species.

There is such a place. There are several of them, in fact, in different parts of the world. Among them are the N. I. Vavilov Gene Bank in the U.S.S.R., and the National Seed Storage Laboratory at Fort Collins, Colorado. Their existence is concrete, although litle-known, evidence of the extent to which some aspects of the evolutionary process are already being managed by public agencies. They have to do with the second part of the global biological transition which is now taking place.

The purpose of the gene banks is to preserve genetic diversity within species. Every species of plant or animal life has its own gene pool, representing all its different varieties. Some species have great genetic diversity, and some very little. The more diversity a species has, the greater its common stock of genetic information: Some varieties may possess special qualities (such as resistance to a given disease or adaptability to a given climate) that others lack. New plant diseases are forever evolving, and the species with greater diversity have a larger arsenal of defenses.

The maintenance of genetic diversity is respectably within the realm of public policy—no right-wing legions march to get government out of the gene pool—but at the same time it is not an issue about which much is heard. The federal laws and programs which make up U.S. genetic resource policy were shaped in response to the expressed needs of a small number of organizations, chiefly seed companies and food processors. As a counterpoint to this prevailing group of special interests there are a few dissidents who believe the official policy is inadequate and is permitting—even encouraging—an alarming "erosion" of genetic resources. The great majority of people in the United States and the rest of the world neither know nor care about gene resource policy, although it could reasonably be argued that the diminution of genetic variety in the world's major food crops is a matter of more immediate concern to our daily well-being than the arcane bits of economic data—such as fluctuations in the money supply—about which informed people feel obliged to have knowledge and opinions.

All the world's major food crops derive originally from a few regions of natural genetic diversity. These are the Vavilov centers, the Earth's erogenous zones. Most are in tropical climes where evolution flourished during the Ice Age while the present temperate zones were frozen.[5] Most of them, in fact, are in what we now call the Third World. This means that the economically and industrially underdeveloped nations of the world are "gene-rich"; they have a great diversity of species and subspecies, while the developed nations are "gene-poor". There may be immense *populations* of certain plants or animals in the nations of the temperate zones, but there is no corresponding diversity of species and subspecies. The tropical zones have more native plant and insect species than the scientists have ever been able to count, and an equally impressive range of higher life forms. Costa Rica alone has 850 different species of birds—more than the entire United States and Canada combined. A bit north of Costa Rica is the Mexico-Guatemala Vavilov center, where corn was first cultivated and where many commercial crop plants—including cacao, tobacco, sisal, pumpkin, squash, papaya, pineapple, pecan, various kinds of peppers, and the common bean which is a major food staple for most of Latin America—once grew wild. Scientists are not sure of the precise places of origin, since extensive seed-trading was already going on among the agriculturally sophisticated Indian civilizations thousands of years before the first Europeans arrived.

By contrast the United States, although one of the world's major food exporters, has no major native food plants. Of the thousand or so crops harvested in North America, there are only a handful—among them Jerusalem artichokes, cranberries, and sunflowers—that originated here.[6] The rest are immigrants. All the plants that people depend on for food are well-traveled. Some of them—rice, for example—have been on the move for thousands of years. Other movements are of more recent date, such as the introduction of tomatoes and potatoes into Europe by the Spanish who had discovered them in South America.

When plants travel and are cultivated, they are selectively bred over time to many regional variations. Also, many wild native varieties survive in the areas where they originated. This adds up to much genetic diversity, a great wealth of information.

In recent years, however, there has been a striking shrinkage of genetic diversity within many of the major crop plants. This genetic erosion, as it is called, has two causes: One is standardization, the other is alteration or destruction of ecosystems in areas of genetic diversity.

Standardization is characteristic of modern agribusiness. In ancient India, over 5500 varieties of rice were cultivated.[7] In the Mexico-Guatemala highlands where corn was first cultivated, there are different varieties for different alititudes, different hillsides, different families.[8] But in the present-day United States an entire national crop may grow from a few strains. American farmers grow only three kinds of millet, for example, two kinds of peas, four varieties of potatoes.[9] This is a biological situation that exists within a framework of politics and economics—as do more biological situations than we generally suspect. In this case the political framework is provided by the Plant Variety Protection Acts, which established the legal conditions for the patenting of plant varieties. The economic framework is a booming seed industry which is protected by the patenting laws. Once a rurally-based group of family-owned firms, the seed companies have become a hot item in transnational business.

The industry is now dominated by large firms such as DuPont, Sandoz, Ciba-Geigy, Monsanto, Atlantic-Richfield and Occidental Petroleum. More than 60 major seed companies were acquired by multinational conglomerates between 1972 and 1982; Royal Dutch-Shell alone now owns more than 30 American and European seed companies.[10]

One of the major arguments on behalf of patenting is that it spurs research and development. The seed industry is investing millions in new technologies, such as encapsulated seeds that contain chemical fertilizers, pesticides, fungicides and herbicides—all in a single package that is popped into the ground at seeding time. The multinationals are also marketing hybrid varieties that are produced with painstaking care in such places as Southeast Asia and South America, where cheap labor is available for the delicate and exhausting work of brushing pollen from the stamen of one plant onto the ovule of another—work so demanding that in some cases workers can put in only two-hour shifts.

[72]

Other Western nations have their own seed-patent laws, and there is an International Union for the Protection of New Varieties of Plants that coordinates plant patenting laws worldwide. In some countries it is even illegal (punishable by a fine of 400 Pounds Sterling in Great Britain) to plant varieties not listed in the official seed catalog.[11] The consequence is one that does not exactly bear out the stated intent of the Plant Variety Protection Acts: The number of newly-minted patented varieties increases, but overall the gene pool diminishes. Three quarters of the vegetable varieties currently grown in Europe will have disappeared by the end of the century, and a comparable thinning of the genetic ranks is taking place all over the world. It is a major development in the history of agriculture, a remarkable global standardization. Pat Roy Mooney, a Canadian agricultural activist, writes:

> In the spring of 1983 a Canadian prairie gardener planted Nantes and Chantenay carrots . . . and so did another gardener in the highlands of Kenya. Across Africa, Congolese farmers were weeding their Bintje potatoes just as Swedish farmers were planting theirs. Palmetto soybeans were thrusting into the hot sunlight of Malaysia and curling against the night cool of Rwanda. A Philippines-bred rice, IR-8, was in cultivation from Taiwan to Benin. A Mexican wheat, Pitic 62, was being seeded from Canada to Cyprus, and a German sugarbeet was awaiting harvest in Chile.[12]

Mooney, who has emerged in recent years as the leading gadfly of the international seed industry, contends that there is relatively little difference among many of the brands that are patented and marketed as "new" strains.

[73]

The seed companies, he says, are in the habit of bringing out new models which are not noticeably different from those of the previous year or those of their competitors—"chrome and tailfin" plant breeding, he calls it.

However large a role patenting may play, it is not the whole story; there are other forces that favor agricultural standardization. Mechanization is one: Food processing machinery demands certain kinds of crops, such as the famous "tough tomato"—the squarish, hard, thick-skinned and juiceless variety developed by botanists at the University of California at Davis for its ability to be handled by modern harvesting machinery (developed at the same institution) without being turned into tomato juice in the processs. The "green revolution" illustrates another: Although the wheat and rice varieties identified with it are in the public domain, their availability wooed farmers in many parts of the world away from the crops they had previously grown. It is a matter of plain competition: There is a selection process of a non-Darwinian sort which turns farmers toward new varieties, patented or not, that they believe superior to old ones. One geneticist says: "It's true that primitive varieties are disappearing throughout the world, but not because of biotech, scientists or even seed companies. Given the option, farmers choose the varieties that increase the amount of crop they have to sell and thus improve their standard of living. The real bogeyman is the marketplace: governments and individuals expressing their demands for more productive crops."[13]

Yet another part of the picture is the rapid modernization of the seed industry. There was a time—around the turn of the century—when a seed company's catalog might contain six densely-spaced pages of varieties of beans. Such folksy inefficiency comes to an end when the companies are taken over by multinationals. Lists are culled, many varieties are dropped. Each such marketing decision, made in a modern office, requiring only a few touches of the computer keyboard, is a small piece of directed evolution. As one observer puts it: "Whenever a variety is dropped from commercial availability—unless an individual or seed bank decides to make a concerted effort to keep [it] alive—it is on the road to extinction."[14]

Different observers come up with conflicting interpretations of why the astounding genetic diversity created over the centuries by local farmers is disappearing—there is much argument about how much of a role patenting plays—but they all agree that it is disappearing.

Genetic diversity is being reduced in both the developed world and the Third World, in the gene-poor nations and the gene-rich. In the Central American highlands where countless varieties of corn once grew, young farmers are turning to modern hybrids. One biologist encountered thousands of varieties of flax growing on the Cilician plain of Turkey in the 1940s; he returned to the same area twenty years later to find that they had all been displaced by a single variety—imported from Argentina.[15]

Something quite similar is happening with domesticated animals. Although there have never been local variations of domesticated animals in numbers to compare with those of crop plants, there is today a strong trend toward global standardization of them—spurred by the rapidly increasing reliance on artificial insemination and related breeding technologies.

And so a major change is taking place in the genetic condition of the living things most closely connected to the human species, and it is virtually unnoticed by the press or political leaders. All the people who have any knowledge of the matter or who hold any opinion about it—right, left or center—could probably be assembled on a football field, leaving the stadium empty.

Genetic Technology

SPECIES extinction and genetic erosion are both examples of the Lilliput effect: They are large-scale biological alterations caused, mainly inadvertently, by human actions. The third part of the new biological message, however, is somewhat different. It is the result of slow and deliberate scientific progress by the intellectual heirs of Darwin and Mendel, and it is transacting its business at the smallest microscopic levels of life. Yet it is an inseparable part of the genetic reality of the modern world, and a part that must be understood in relation to the others as people begin to think about evolutionary policy.

Molecular biology has been making great strides in recent decades, since the famous breakthrough that revealed the double helix structure of the DNA molecule, and scientists are rapidly gaining more and more knowledge about the inner workings of the genes. The symbolic information system is discovering in ever more precise detail how the genetic information system works, and is becoming capable of directly altering the contents of the genetic message—another evolution of evolution.

The life processes of every organism are carried out according to the directions contained in the DNA that it inherits, and—although we pay less attention to this—all higher organisms depend on things produced by the genetic ingenuity of other organisms. Every organism is a chemical factory, producing compounds that are essential to its own biochemical processes and also to those of other living things. A natural ecosystem is a felicitous interaction of different information systems directing organisms to produce things that nourish other organisms.

The human species from a very early stage of its evolution displayed an uncommon ability to appropriate not only biochemical compounds—foods and medicines—but also fancier items produced from the genetic information of other organism—the furs of animals, for example—and made a great evolutionary stride in moving from hunting and gathering into agriculture: domesticating animals, planting and harvesting grains. This greatly improved the ability of humans to borrow from the information of other species, detoured the evolutionary development of the domesticated species, and also (as we noted in the previous chapter) changed whole ecosystems: Many regions became specialists, supporting fields of grain or herds of sheep instead of their former mixture of species. The emergence of agriculture—the original biotechnology—is often equated with the emergence of civilization itself, linked to the building of cities and the creation of more complex forms of social organization.

Humans developed other biotechnologies such as fermentation to produce bread and alcoholic beverages, and became increasingly skillful at selective breeding to control the genetic information passed along by domesticated animals and food crops. The new biotechnologies are not a departure from the general direction of human evolution— but they are a colossal forward stride, and their appearance marks a transition as great as the beginning of agriculture or the Industrial Revolution. We are now in the early stages of a Biological Revolution.

The Industrial Revolution was a transformation of the means of production; machinery was a part of it but not the whole, since the patterns of social organization that accompanied it were as central to the process as the new technologies. It had, among its many far-reaching economic, ecological and political consequences, the effect of producing many new human interventions in nature. The Biological Revolution is yet another escalation of human intervention in nature, and will have among its consequences new methods of production. Both the Industrial and the Biological Revolutions are rapid changes of pace in things that people had been doing already: in the first instance, manufacturing goods; in the second, manipulating evolution.

The new biotechnologies—the plural form is more accurate—are a complex and fast-moving group of scientific discoveries and technical accomplishments. The one that gets the most attention—often erroneously taken to be the whole of modern biotechnology—is genetic engineering or gene-splicing. This, however, is only a part of a larger repertoire of procedures that is affecting the entire scientific discipline of biology. When we talk about the new biotechnologies we are not talking about a few super-scientists and a few industries that use their discoveries; we are talking about a scientific revolution that is having its effect in every laboratory and classroom. The discoveries and methods associated with biotechnology have changed *all* of biology.

I don't propose to attempt an extensive description of the new biotechnologies in this chapter; several good introductory books—not to mention several bad ones—are available, and the reader who wants greater technical detail would do well to read an explanation written by someone with a steadier grip on the science than my own.[16] But I do want to review some of the major approaches briefly—partly in order to assemble a picture of the evolutionary and political power they bring into the world, and partly because some clarity about what is being done makes it easier to avoid the hokum that so persistently stalks this subject.

Gene-splicing arises logically out of recent developments in the science of molecular biology. Once it became understood that genetic information consists of certain chemical compounds arranged in a certain way, it became *theoretically* possible to move such information from one organism to another—and even from one species to another, since, at the molecular level, all life is made up of the same chemicals and structured according to the same architecture. This is a discovery that surely would have spoiled the morning for Bishop Wilberforce, since it says that the fundamental molecular chemistry of human beings is the same as that of apes—and of mushrooms, too, as a matter of fact.

The word "theoretically" is important here, because the DNA molecule remains a thing of stunning complexity even after its basic organizational structure stands revealed. New practical applications of gene-splicing are being developed every day, but there is still a tremendous amount to be learned; the revolution has scarcely begun.

The life form that has been the most "engineered", the minute workhorse of biotechnology that became as important a part of the human adventure as dogs and wheat and *Drosophila* and laboratory mice, is the intestinal bacterium *E. coli*. And the major tool of bio-engineering is the restriction enzyme. Scientists have discovered some 350 enzymes that are capable of cutting into a DNA molecule at specific points along its chain of genetic information. On the basis of this it became possible to splice new genetic information into *E. coli*, turning each bacterium into a small factory which produces some kind of bio-chemical its evolutionary history had never taught it to make—such as human insulin and human growth hormone, to name two of the first commercial products of gene-splicing.

Let us take a look at a few interesting points about these early applications.

Note, first of all, that they follow from and improve upon other techniques for obtaining similar biochemicals—techniques that were in themselves elaborate manipulations of human and animal biochemistry. Insulin for human use has for some time been obtained from butchered pigs and cattle, whose insulin is chemically close enough to our own that in the human body it does a satisfactory job of controlling levels of blood sugar—satisfactory but not perfect, since the minor chemical difference causes reactions in some patients, and there is always the danger of impurities. Insulin produced by genetic engineering is identical to the chemical produced in the human pancreas, and free of impurities. Human growth hormone had been obtained from the pituitary glands of dead people. The procedure was expensive, the supply limited, and, again, there was the danger of impurities.

Note, second, that these biochemicals produce significant improvements in the quality of life for certain people who were born with genetic deficiencies and who would live less satisfying lives without it: Insulin enables diabetics to live relatively normal lives, growth hormone enables children who would otherwise be dwarves to grow to normal height. At the same time, the use of any such remedy also constitutes an intervention in human genetic evolution: It affects the individual's chances of surviving, reproducing, and passing his or her genetic information along to future generations. This is true whether the chemical is produced through genetic engineering or not. But it is a point worth keeping in mind lest one is temped to resolve the moral and political issues by taking the deceptively simple position that nothing should be done that intervenes in human evolution. If there is to be no such intervention, then diabetics should be deprived of insulin and required to die natural deaths or at least sterilized—which would be an intervention. Also, we should remember that the material is capable of being used in ways not quite the same as what the manufacturers intended. Growth hormone can not only turn a dwarf into a normal-sized person; it can turn a short person into a tall one, an average-sized one into somebody about the right size for a lineman in professional football. Again, this was true before the hormone was being manufactured by biotechnology—but it is obviously a more critical question as availability increases.

Note, third, that even these rather primitive manipulations of genetic material operate on a new plateau of evolutionary intervention. It is one thing for human beings to breed selectively, slowly bringing out this or that characteristic in some life form; it is something quite different to create a new organism with new abilities *that do not come out of the evolutionary heritage of its own species.* It means that the concept of a species which was fundamental to Darwinian and post-Darwinian thought—of a species as a distinct life form which does not crossbreed with another species, and whose characteristics have been developed as adaptation to its natural environment—is no longer adequate to all cases; it is certainly not adequate to describe a bacterium that produces human insulin.

[81]

Most of the gene-splicing accomplishments thus far have been down around the lower levels of the Great Chain of Being—but nevertheless this form of biotechnology has brought millions of new organisms into the world and has affected the lives—and evolutionary futures—of many plants and animals and people. And meanwhile other biotechnological methods are developing rapidly.

One technique is the fusion of two kinds of animal cells to produce a hybrid cell with new and unique properties. In the most important experiments of this sort, an antibody-producing spleen cell is combined with a rapidly-multiplying cancer cell. The result is a cell that reproduces itself prolifically and produces antibodies. The antibodies can be used to combat leukemic blood cells, to diagnose cancer and other diseases, possibly to develop a new kind of contraceptive with antibodies specific to the proteins in human sperm—even specific to female or male chromosomes, thus providing a precise method of predetermining a child's sex,[17] and as a tool to work jointly with recombinant DNA technology to lay the basis for a revolution in immunology.

Immunization is one of the human species' most valuable biotechnologies, one that was being successfully practiced before people understood how it really worked. Its history in the Western world dates back to 1796, the year the English country doctor Edward Jenner decided to check out the folk belief that milkmaids became immune to smallpox because they contracted the similar but much less deadly cowpox. Operating in a fashion that would blow the mind of a modern food and drug bureaucrat, Jenner inoculated an eight-year-old boy with pus from a cowpox-infected milkmaid and then exposed the boy to smallpox. The boy did not contract smallpox, and a new phase of intervention in nature began.

What happens when such a material is introduced into the body is, as one writer puts it, "a sort of teaching session": Exposure to a closely related but less virulent microbe, or to the dead virulent microbe, teaches the body how to deal with that particular invader.[18]

Molecular biology has made it increasingly clear how this educational process takes place. Bacteria, viruses and other invaders contain substances called antigens whose presence triggers a chemical response in the body, causing it to produce antibodies which attack the antigen and neutralize it. It takes a while for this response to mobilize itself—for the body to learn what to do—and during this lag period the individual may suffer or die from the disease. A vaccine overcomes that delay by teaching the body how to recognize the invader in advance. There are different ways of doing this—injecting a weakened form of the disease bacterium (tuberculosis vaccine), injecting inactivated virus (Salk polio vaccine), injecting treated forms of the toxins from the disease organism (tetanus vaccine). Monoclonal antibody technology in combination with gene-splicing—using the ever-popular *E. coli* or some other bacterium to manufacture the vaccine—created new research methods for studying how antigens and antibodies work, vastly improved ability to diagnose disease, and produced ways of teaching the bodies of human beings and animals how to overcome their ancient enemies. If there were nothing more to the Biological Revolution than the advances in immunology, this alone would constitute a major development in global evolution—not only affecting the chances of survival of millions of human beings but also immensely improving the prospects for many species of domestic animals to survive and breed in hostile ecosystems.

Cell fusion work (somewhat similar to that done with animal cells to produce monoclonal antibodies) is being done extensively with plant cells. The outer walls of the cells are dissolved, and the two naked cells—called pro-toplasts—are then combined to form a single new cell which can, with careful nurturing in hormone solutions, be persuaded to grow into a new plant. Some cells of different plant species have been combined this way—the best known being an interesting but agriculturally un-productive potato-tomato hybrid called a "pomato".

The ability to grow whole plants from cells—either protoplasts or cells from a single plant—is one of the most powerful tools of the new agricultural high tech-nology. It increases the speed and range of experimentation. Cloning, the lurid subject of genetic fiction, is commonly practiced by plant researchers who can take a plant cell and culture it into full regeneration to produce a new plant which is a faithful genetic copy of the original.[19] This adds great precision to some lines of research—it becomes possible to grow identical plants in different cli-mates and measure the results with unprecedented effi-ciency—and also enables growers to plant entire crops of a superior individual. It is as though a horse breeder, freed from the uncertainties of sexual reproduction, could produce a whole stable of Man O' Wars. This method is already producing crops, and has been for some time. A research team at Unilever in England developed a tissue-culture method of producing clonal palm trees which were sent to Malaysia as small bare-root plants in 1976 and were bearing fruit a couple of years later—a latter-day high-tech episode in the British Empire's long saga of colonial ecosystem transformation.[20] The likely prospect is that fields of identical plants will become commonplace as the technology advances. One of the most promising commercial products so far is the somatic embryo encapsulation—the "synthetic seed", a small quantity of genetic material enclosed in an artificial polymer coat. These produce uniform, identical plants, with no Mendelian eccentricities; and the seed can be designed to contain not only genetic information but herbicides, pesticides, and fertilizer.

There are several other things that can be done with cell- and tissue-culture technology. One line of experimentation has been in the direction of developing crops that will grow in salty soil. A culture of oat cells, for example, can be doused with heavy solutions of salt. Most die, but the survivors with high salt tolerance are cloned and regenerated into salt-resistant plants. At the International Rice Research Institute in the Philippines, researchers are working on varities of rice that will tolerate the high salt and aluminum soils found in parts of Southeast Asia. Scientists can search for mutants in this manner; they can also create them by using chemicals, x-rays, etc. This, again, is not entirely new; "conventional" plant-breeding biotechnology is already adept at inducing mutation. But with cell or tissue cultures it becomes possible to experiment with many thousands of individual plants in a small laboratory, and to do it much more rapidly.

All of this adds up to a technological revolution that is causing profound changes in plant breeding even though actual gene-splicing of food plants is still at a very early stage. It is a revolution that overlaps with conventional plant-breeding and is not separable from it. There is much commuting between the laboratories and the fields as the new creations are grown and tested. Molecular biology is accelerating plant breeding, and it is also accelerating evolution as it speeds up the creation and discovery of mutations, the production of new plant varieties, and the movement of genetic information about the world.

A similar revolution is taking place in animal breeding, as new biological knowledge revolutionizes the art and science of selectively guiding the evolution of domesticated species. In dairy farming, the day when farmers transported their cows on conjugal visits to neighboring bulls is long gone. The technology of artificial insemination has taken over, and bull semen is now a familiar commodity of international commerce. Embryo transfer is also widely used: The embryos from a prize cow are removed, frozen, stored, and shipped here and there to be brought to life inside surrogate mothers in another state or another country. Scientists are working on other manipulations of the reproductive process: *in vitro* fertilization, inducing multiple births, even—in a process somewhat similar to the cloning of plants—dissociating and developing cells from an embryo so that it results in not one animal but several, genetically identical.

These various methods are parts of a fast-moving scientific revolution that is both conceptual—changes in how people see and understand genetic information—and technical. The technology is moving fast, and more breakthroughs can be expected. One of the most promising fields is "protein engineering": Where the first products of recombinant DNA were biochemicals found in nature— such as human insulin—a technique called "site-directed mutagenisis" allows scientists to create proteins that have new structures and new properties.

[86]

The Biological Jet Set

THE FOURTH factor in the current biological transition is the movement of life forms about the globe.

As the scientists transfer microscopic genetic information from one organism to another, other people transfer other kinds of genetic information—such as seeds, cuttings, frozen semen, frozen embryos, living plants and animals—from one continent to another. It is curious that, while the increased global mobility of people is an obvious and generally accepted reality, so little attention is paid to the inescapable fact that people are not the only things doing the traveling—that the mobility of plants and animals is increasing also, and that this constitutes another large (and irreversible) change in the world's biological condition.

Like the other processes involved in the current global genetic transition, the movement of nonhuman life forms by humans has been going on for a long time. The first such movements were probably accidental transplants, much like the transplantation of European grasses to California by the Spaniards. But with the beginning of agriculture—the first biotechnology—transplantation became systematic and deliberate.

Recombinant DNA technology, operating at the molecular level, moves genetic information from one cell to another and—if successful—the gene "expresses" and the cell carries out the chemical process for which it has received instructions. Agriculture brings genetic information into a new ecosystem and—if successful—gets it to grow and reproduce. Agricultural transplantations, whether of plants or animals, always have secondary effects: Pests come along for the ride, predators and ecological rivals have to be forcefully combated, and the world changes in small ways or large. In agriculture, human beings have been moving species around the globe and altering ecosystems for thousands of years. Today the amount of such world travel is on the rise.

Botanists have often noted that there are a great many more edible plants in the world than are commonly used, and some of them are now systematically seeking out promising plants to be grown and eaten in other places. Little-known grains such as amaranth may come to be cultivated in many parts of the world, a new agriculture and a new source of nutrition.

Paralleling this interest in little-known food plants is a booming appetite in developed nations for plants that have long been favorites in other countries. American farmers and grocery dealers are suddenly discovering the merits of mamey, the national fruit of Cuba, lychee and longan from China; carambola from Southeast Asia. Growers in Florida are reported to be cutting down citrus trees and putting in jakfruit—another native of Southeast Asia, which produces individual fruits that weigh as much as 60 pounds.

Part of the movement of plants is, as it has always been, incidental to other migrations: The human species is currently engaged in what some demographers believe may be the largest global migration of all time—moving from depleted rural areas to the cities, from the Third World to Europe and North America. As people move they bring their traditional foods—and some of them open restaurants—and the American ecosystems, which are the true melting pots, become more cosmopolitan than ever. The *Smithsonian* reports: "Vietnamese are growing lemongrass; Indian immigrants are tending curry plants and ivy gourds; Cubans are producing malanga, bonaito, and calabaza; and West Indians are raising dasheen and pigeon peas."[21] As people move they carry fruits, vegetables, and seeds—and often, without meaning to, insects or larvae. The growing world trade in food also provides transportation for various pests, and so do other kinds of commerce; in California there has recently been concern about gypsy moths sneaking into the state aboard Christmas trees from Oregon.

Animal movement is increasing also: the transfer of rare animals to zoos, the various forms of transportation connected with the new technologies of animal breeding. Paralleling the interest in exotic plants is an interest in animals not previously domesticated that might be of agricultural value.

There is hardly any development in biology or agriculture that does not involve transporting genetic information from one place to another. In response to concern about depletion of genetic resources, for example, the scientists conscientiously travel to the centers of diversity to gather samples. The laboratories and gene storage centers acquire and exchange material as they build up their collections. Even efforts to "restore" ecosystems send scientists shopping about the globe in search of useful material. Restoration often requires ingenious substitution if an ecosystem has been extensively damaged. When the federal government set out to repair the destruction of the Dust Bowl disaster of the 1930s, the native grasses failed to take hold in the depleted soil and grasses from Africa came to the rescue. Similarly, reforestation projects commonly resort to planting trees from other regions (or other continents) that commend themselves for various qualities such as fast growth. Inevitably, as data storage and exchange becomes easier, people with a certain task in mind will find it possible to select from a global inventory.

The new biotechnologies of livestock reproduction add another dimension to this global movement by making it possible for breeders to ship frozen semen and embryos about the world nearly as easily as they can ship plant seeds. Embryos do not, like live animals, carry diseases and parasites with them, and their small size makes shipping costs attractive. One scientist working in this field boasts that "You can ship 2,000 cows under your airplane seat."[22]

Another part of the mass migration of life forms now underway is largely illegal—the international trade in rare and exotic pets, including specimens of species that are close to extinction.

All these put together add up to a lot of life forms moving from one place to another, a vast pattern of human interventions in evolution. The capture of rare animals hastens their extinction in their native habitat. Introduction of animals and plants often changes ecosystems as happened in California when the European grass crowded the native varieties out of their econiche. The deliberate introduction of new agricultural crops has similar impacts. Conversely, removal of large numbers of a species such as a key predator may disturb the balance of the ecosystem from which they are taken. As a result of such interventions, ecosystems everywhere undergo extensive changes; they also come to resemble one another as exotic species appear among the natives. New connections are made—actions taken that it would be impossible to undo—and the world becomes a biosphere in a way it has never been before.

Kubernetes

I HAVE described the present evolutionary transition as shooting the rapids. Such metaphors are never exact, of course, but politics depends heavily on metaphors and myths. They give shape and a certain human scale to our information, and are especially helpful in those situations— more common than we like to believe—where we must act on the basis of incomplete data.

When you are steering a vessel—let us say a raft plunging down a fast-flowing river—you are partly in control, partly out of control; the situation demands its own special kind of ingenuity and skill. There are some things you cannot do: You cannot, even if the voyage is turning out to be not to your liking, paddle back upstream to where you started from. Neither can you plan out precisely what you are going to do at each point along the way ahead. You take the rapids and bends and eddies as they come. But you cannot merely relax and float downstream; river runners who try that end up wet at best and often dead, their vessels in tatters on the rocks. Skill is important; the more you know about the ways of rivers and rafts, the better. Learning is central; you constantly adjust your course in reponse to visual and kinetic information, and you get better at it as you proceed.

In the late 1940s, when the Information Revolution was just getting underway, the word *cybernetics* was invented. It came from the Greek word *kubernetes*, which means steersman or helmsman. Cybernetics became a general designation for the whole field of communication and control theory, relating to both mechanical and animal intelligence. The word was chosen to call attention to the importance of feedback; it signifies control, of course, in the image of the helmsman with his hand on the tiller— but Norbert Weiner, who coined the term, was more interested in calling attention to the *process* involved. The helmsman is constantly correcting his course, taking in several kinds of information and acting upon it and then adjusting again in response to whatever has resulted from the previous action. This process became the symbol for all the actions living things perform to survive in nature and all the feats that new computers and servo-mechanisms could be designed to do.

As it happens, *kubernetes* is also the root of the the English word "govern". That is something worth keeping in mind, since over the past few decades people have tended to think of a government as something like a huge factory, churning out laws and regulations in mindless response to "inputs" from the public and organized interest groups. The image of the helmsman offers a different way of looking at governance—especially when attention is directed to the role of feedback: The helmsman does not dominate either the vessel or the elements, but interacts with them. We see governance as something more than control; it is also learning. Furthermore, we see a government—any government—not as a huge factory standing stolidly on its ground, but as something in motion, swept along through history.

The matters we have described in this chapter are definitely in motion, flowing swiftly as any river. None of them is about to be halted or reversed: Even the most hopeful naturalists know that thousands of species will be lost during the present decades of extinction; there is a similar inertia to genetic erosion, a global pattern of cause and effect that can be moderated but not arrested. Furthermore—and this is an aspect of the situation which we have not yet had time to think about—preservation of a species or a variety does not bring evolution to a halt, or even put it on hold, buts sets in motion new patterns of intervention. The new biotechnologies represent a different kind of change, an ongoing explosion of new knowledge; the movement of plant and animal life has its own momentum, its own logic, and its own economy. Everywhere we look in the world are unfolding sequences of human intervention.

We cannot govern without constantly applying the *kubernetes* process of seeking feedback and altering course, but I do not mean to suggest that it is a formula which, once applied, solves the problem. It will be as difficult to apply as are any of the other master principles of governance—like separation of powers—that are already part of our political culture. Information about what may result from a given line of action is not always available, and we do not have well-established institutional practices for using the information we have. Governance decisions are always made on the basis of less than complete information—that is the only kind of information there is— and usually with much disagreement about what the facts are and what they mean. We have a lot to learn about information; this should become apparent as we survey some recent and current examples of evolutionary governance in action.

[4]

Biopolitics

ALTHOUGH few people are aware of the great genetic transition that is now taking place—do not comprehend it as a systemic pattern of global change—many isolated aspects of the transition have already surfaced as political issues. These issues are the beginnings of a shift from environmentalism to biopolitics—to a larger frame of reference that includes such concerns as the general problem of extinction (not just the loss of certain species), genetic erosion, and regulation of the new biotechnologies.

Some of these biopolitical issues are products of the Industrial Revolution in its late stages; some are products of the Biological Revolution in its early stages. We are in a time of political as well as biological transition, and—since we lack a general and publicly-articulated idea of the biological changes—we have not really begun to consider the possibility that we are dealing with a new class of political problems.

The changes in methods of production that began to take place in England about two centuries ago surely did not seem to anyone at the time to constitute a watershed event in the history of Western society; they were merely a few innovations in machinery and organization, diverse happenings with no apparent interconnection or long-range political import. The Industrial Revolution stole upon England unawares; its scope and meaning were not comprehended even when it had become the most conspicuous thing on the landscape. But, as we can see from this side of history, it was an enormous and powerful force that would roll through England, leap to the European Continent and North America, and in time reach every corner of the world. It was not just an event, but the beginning of a series of events of which we have yet to see an end—a continuous process of innovation. It was a change in much more than methods of production; one of its historians calls it "the most fundamental transformation of human life in the history of the world recorded in written documents."[1]

It had ecological consequences: One of the first great industries, textiles, was dependent for its raw material on the cotton plantations of the American southern states, where huge artificial ecosystems had been carved out of the land, planted with cotton (various strains native to Egypt, Asia, Mexico, and South America), and worked by human beings transplanted from Africa.

It had economic consequences: It hastened the transition to a money economy, brought new economic institutions into being and shaped human consciousness toward the view of all things—including human labor—as marketable commodities.

[95]

It had social consequences: It reordered the class system, disrupted old institutions and folkways, and set the patterns for new forms of interaction and organization.

And it had political consequences: It transformed the nation-state, gave birth to new laws and regulations and governmental structures, formed the basis for modern political parties, and brought forth new political ideologies.

Contemporary political ideologies are different sets of ideas about how to deal with the Industrial Revolution. Basically they come in two packages. One ideological group consists of the "free market" theories which hold that the mechanism of free trade is essentially self-regulating; its aim is to separate the economy from society. The second set of ideas attempts to impose social guidance of some sort—regulation, planning, transfer payments—upon the economic system in the name of public interest. Karl Polanyi, one of the great historians of the Industrial Revolution, insisted that collectivism on the whole never represented a single ideology or movement so much as a series of *ad hoc* responses to situations in which society was imperiled by the market.[2] Socialism of course is a coherent ideological movement, but many of the most significant collectivist policies enacted in the past—Bismarck's adoption of social security is the classic example—were attempts to outflank socialism by redressing injustices of the market system in order to make socialist solutions less attractive to the public.

The ideological orientations born out of the Industrial Revolution continue to predominate in a world that is now being forced to deal with an entirely new set of problems. However, this situation will problably not continue for very long. We have seen some attempts to form new ideologies and movements appropriate to the environmental stage, and as we survey reactions to the present period of biological instability we may catch glimpses of perspectives that might more correctly be called biopolitical.

Although the idea of human responsibility for evolution is a novel one, especially in political circles, we have already progressed a considerable distance into the uncharted seas of biopolitics. There are laws and regulations pertaining to every one of the four aspects of global genetic change mentioned in the foregoing chapter, and issues of evolutionary governance are being disputed in capitols and courthouses around the world. For the most part these fit well within the mode of politics as we have known it, although sometimes the old language fails: When that happens, the policymakers and the interest groups and the activists find themselves in a position rather like that of characters in an animated cartoon who have run off the edge of the cliff but do not know until they look down that the familiar solid ground is no longer beneath them.

Let us look at some of the issues and policies that have emerged around each of the four aspects of biological change that I have identified—species extinction, genetic erosion, biotechnology and species movement.

Protecting Endangered Species

THERE IS a long history of isolated federal and state policies that included some protection of wild species— park programs and hunting and fishing regulations, for example—but it was not until 1966 that the first step was taken toward an explicit national policy. In 1966 Senator Karl Mundt of South Dakota introduced a bill to create an Endangered Species Bureau in the Department of the

Interior. The bill's stated purpose was to "bring endangered species in out of the wild and attempt to raise them in captivity." It passed, but along the way it generated some examples of the ponderous humor that frequently arises in connection with this subject. Mundt's colleagues dubbed it the "dickey-bird bill of 1966."

The dickey-bird bill did not do any great amount of good to endangered species in the United States, but it didn't make any enemies for its cause, and in 1973, at the height of the environmental binge, Congress passed the Endangered Species Act. This bill—which was in many ways a twin of the National Environmental Policy Act—stated a general policy that "all Federal departments and agencies shall seek to conserve endangered species and threatened species." Like NEPA it was a sleeper; it passed without much opposition and, in fact, without much comprehension of how difficult it would be to carry out its mandates.

The Endangered Species Act was a political innovation as momentous in its way as the Magna Carta. It is a remarkable event, if you stop to think about it, when a group of human beings agree that the survival and extinction of species are not to be left to Darwinian roulette, but will also be governed by public policy. The bill passed chiefly because the legislators did *not* stop to think about it. Certainly they did not consider that, since evolution and polity and economy are inseparable, regulating evolution might also involve some diversion of the line of march of economic progress.

But soon the confrontations began. In the state of Maine there was a confrontation between a dam and a small plant called the Furbish lousewort. In Tennessee there was a confrontation between a dam and a fish called the snail darter, a tiny creature that had been numerous when the waters of the Tennessee Valley were free-flowing systems. The snail darter soon became the star of the production, even though it was not really what the argument was about; there had already been local opposition to the Tellico Dam. Nevertheless, when the fish entered the picture it became the chief weapon of the anti-dam activists. They got the Secretary of the Interior to designate the snail darter an endangered species and to set aside 17 miles of the Little Tennessee River as "threatened habitat" essential to its survival. This opened the way for a lawsuit that won an injunction against the Tennessee Valley Authority. The U.S. Supreme Court upheld the injunction, ruling that if Congress wanted the dam built it would have to exempt the project from the Endangered Species Act. A huge Congressional debate ensued, with some legislators quoting from the Bible as authority for human dominion in such matters. Finally Congress passed, and President Jimmy Carter signed, a bill exempting the Tellico project from "any law that might hinder construction"— not mentioning the Endangered Species Act specifically. In 1978, Congress also passed some amendments to weaken the act—making it more difficult to get "endangered" or "threatened" designation and limiting the federal commitment in other ways. But the law is still on the books— and the snail darter, having been transplanted to other waters, survives also.

Even when people agree that a given species ought to be saved from extinction, they often disagree about how to do it; there have been many biopolitical controversies about what *kind* of protection policy should be adopted to save a species. California has been the scene of a long conflict over the giant condor: The Audubon Society favored breeding condors in captivity, looking forward to some future time when they might be safely released. Other environmental groups advocated protecting the habitat so that the birds could have something like a natural life—and feared that a decision to breed in captivity would produce a relaxation of efforts to protect the habitat.

The Audubon strategy won governmental approval, and a Condor Recovery Program was launched, a co-operative effort of the National Audubon Society and the U.S. Fish and Wildlife Service. An early attempt to capture a condor chick to rear in captivity led to the chick's death when it was roughly handled by a scientist attempting to examine it in its nest. Later, however, two chicks were successfully captured and reared in the Los Angeles zoo. Another part of the recovery program called for taking eggs from the nest and hatching them in captivity; this approach is justified in part by the so-called "double clutching" characteristic of the condors and some other birds—when one egg is taken, the female lays a second egg to replace it. The first condor was hatched in the San Diego Zoo in 1983—hatched into the modern world, with the aid of people who used surgical tools to help the chick get free of its tough shell. The chick was bathed in a salt solution, placed in a plastic box to guard it against infection, and fed by a hook-beaked puppet so that it would not imprint on some zookeeper and grow up believing it was a human being.

Some environmentalists protest that a bird so raised is only a facsimile of a giant condor; the zoo side responds that, with the numbers of birds in the wild dwindling to a point where its odds of survival are low and the danger of genetic deterioration from inbreeding is high, breeding in captivity is the only hope of preserving the species. As the population of captive condors grew the population of wild condors dwindled, and zookeepers in Los Angeles and San Diego began to express doubts about reintroducing condors to the wild at all.

There are not only differences of opinion involved here, but differences of interest as well: The conservationists and zookeepers all want to preserve the condors but disagree about how to do it; other people have other plans for the land where the condors nest and no particular commitment to their preservation. The owners of a ranch frequented by wild condor refused to sell it to the U.S. Fish and Wildlife service; they planned to subdivide it and build houses.

I suspect that by the time this book is published the last of the wild condors will be gone, and I am not sanguine about any early re-stocking from the zoos. I have seen the California condors in their native terrain—stood foolhardily atop a mountain in a thunderstorm, unwilling to take my eyes away from those enormous birds circling in the distant grey sky. I had gotten to that place by car, an easy drive up the freeway from Los Angeles. The condor country is heavily traversed by hunters and hikers, close to growing cities. It is hard to imagine a time this side of World War III when California will be much of a home to a giant vulture.

Attempts to preserve endangered life forms are controversial both politically and scientifically. There are divergent views about what constitutes preservation and different technical approaches to the challenge of protecting a species or subspecies on the brink of extinction; often these are new and inadequately tested and thus all the more likely to be disputed. The arguments are intensified by the sense of urgency that conservationists naturally feel when only a pitiful few surviving members of a species remain and a mistake may spell the end to their evolutionary story.

The case of the dusky sparrow illustrates some of the issues involved. This small, black-and-white-feathered subspecies once existed in several places along the East Coast of the United States, but by the 1960s it was surviving in only two habitats: One was Merritt Island in Florida, a site that it shared with the Kennedy Space center. The federal government, whose environmental management policies were not yet guided by the Endangered Species Act, was at the time more concerned about ridding the space center of mosquitos than preserving dusky sparrows, and flooded the marshes in that area. The other site, the St. Johns River a few miles away, became the dusky sparrow's last holdout and was given federal protection in the 1970s; the government spent $2.65 million dollars to purchase the land, and established the St. Johns river refuge. However, calling the area a refuge was not quite enough protection for the marshy region so close to Florida's urbanized Atlantic seaboard, and by 1979 there were only 13 dusky sparrows left—all male. The U.S. Fish and Wildlife Service (the agency charged with the sparrow's evolutionary destiny) decided to try to preserve it in captivity and the remaining birds—by this time only five— were captured and placed in two large cages, specially built and planted with saw grass to simulate their natural marshy habitat, in the Training Zoo at Santa Fe Community College.

The problem that remained was how to preserve a subspecies whose total population consisted of five males. A scientific "recovery team" brought in by the Fish and Wildlife service proposed a crossbreeding strategy, a piece of Mendelian trickery achievable by selectively mating dusky sparrows with females of a closely related subspecies. Under this program a biologist crossed a dusky sparrow with a Scott seaside sparrow and obtained three chicks, one of them with plumage only a bit lighter than the true dusky. The biologist predicted that with five generations of back-crossing he could produce a bird that would be 96.9 percent pure dusky. But the agency's lawyers protested that this was creating a new subspecies, not protecting the old one, and finally it was decided to end the cross-breeding program and keep the remaining dusky sparrows celibate in hopes that a female dusky might be found somewhere. Meanwhile a physiologist at a wildlife research laboratory in Maryland went to work on a procedure to freeze sparrow semen which could be preserved until biological science gets to the point of being able to clone birds from it.[3]

Such sagas seem ludicrous to people who do not worry overmuch about whether some obscure life form disappears, sad to those who do, and primitive to those who believe that we should concentrate on saving ecosystems rather than merely saving species. Once the environment that sustains the life of a given species—such as the California giant condor—has been virtually eliminated, the species itself becomes as vulnerable as a human being whose kidneys no longer function; it is then dependent for its survival on those equivalents of the dialysis machine, the zoo and the wildlife refuge. Consequently, many ecologists now stress not the preservation of species but the value of genetic diversity and the protection of ecosystems. Some American ecosystems—Southern savannas and lowland Hawaiian forest, for example—are already "extinct" and others are on the endangered list.

There are conservation groups who specialize in this field, and a growing body of programs among state and local governments and private organizations that approach the task as one somewhat similar to the preservation of natural landmarks.[4]

As the techniques and the policies of ecosystem/species/subspecies preservation evolve, so does the debate about whether any such preservation efforts are called for at all.

There are different kinds of advocates for protection of wild species. Some people stress compassion for living things, their right to survive, and the mandates that come down from various religious traditions concerning human responsibility for the products of Creation. Other people work from a utilitarian ethic and stress the countless ways that flora and fauna are useful; they often point out, for example, that medical science relies heavily on materials obtained from plants and animals. Not only in medicine but in every aspect of daily life we use materials obtained directly from plants and animals, biochemicals synthesized from those that they have developed for their own survival needs, or "inventions" plagiarized from the vast storehouse of genetic wisdom. Velcro, one of the ubiquitous gadgets of modern life, was developed by a Swiss botanist who had studied the means by which cockelburs fastened themselves so tenaciously to his socks.

Norman Myers, probably the world's foremost advocate of species protection, has in his recent works tended more and more toward emphasizing the utilitarian arguments.[5] His decision is admittedly one of practical politics, based on the recognition that these arguments are the ones most people are prepared to listen to. But Myers also points out that if the utilitarian case is pursued far enough it turns into something larger than a mere defense of exploitation: One begins to see that human life is a web of relationships to other living things.

The human species will have to develop, as part of its own evolutionary progress, a much clearer understanding of the connection between humanity and other forms of life on the planet. As a step in that direction, we would do well to understand that a world which contains many different species is a vast storehouse of genetic information. Every living thing is not only a chemical factory but also a kind of laboratory, which has developed a successful strategy for surviving—and the variety of such strategies, as any student of nature knows, is incredibly wide.

A few years ago a team of Australian zoologists found a frog. It was a remarkable discovery for a couple of reasons: first, that for decades biologists had believed there were no aquatic frogs in Australia; second, that the frog had a reproductive system unlike any other known animal. The female hatches its eggs inside its own stomach. When the young are ready to be born, they emerge fully developed from the mother's mouth. Once in a while one of them appears to be a preemie, and she swallows it until it is ready to try again. Medical scientists immediately took an interest, wondering if the frog's ability to protect its young from its own digestive fluids might hold some secret of use in the treatment of human stomach ulcers.

The current loss of species is a massive loss of genetic information; the destruction of habitat recalls the burning of the great library at Alexandria by Roman soldiers, or the destruction of the records of Indian civilizations in the New World by Spanish soldiers. We do not know precisely what was lost, but we know that its value was not comprehended by those who destroyed it.

[105]

There are good economic and utilitarian reasons for being concerned about the loss of species, but whether the values are utilitarian or aesthetic or religious, they express the beginnings of an awareness that we are living in a different kind of world, one in which the survival or extinction of species results from human action. The mythic theme of Noah and the ark often arises in discussions of this subject. One of Myers' books is entitled *The Sinking Ark*; another book on species preservation is *Building an Ark*; Paul Ehrlich co-authored *Ark II*; another writer speaks of "the Noah principle."[6] In the modern retelling of the story, the flood is a tide of human population growth and technological progress, building and timber-cutting and development; the ark is the world; we are all Noah; and there is no Mount Ararat in sight.

Genes: The Newest and Oldest Resource

THE SUBJECT of genetic erosion raises questions quite similar to those concerning species extinction: whether it matters at all, and how it matters.

One answer invokes the well-known vulnerability of monocultures. When large numbers of people become dependent on a food crop grown from a single strain, a disease which infects it can produce enormous and far-reaching consequences. The Irish potato famine is the classic example: It resulted in untold suffering, two million deaths, a great reduction of the population of Ireland, and a major change in the genetic and cultural makeup of the population of the United States.

Smaller episodes of that sort happen frequently. They do not have the massive consequences of the Irish potato famine—chiefly because most countries have learned the lesson of history and diversified their agricultures—but there are still recurrent plagues on major commercial crops. An outbreak of corn leaf blight destroyed nearly 20 percent of the U.S. corn crop in 1970; a National Academy of Sciences study blamed the epidemic on "a quirk in the technology that had redesigned the corn plants of America until, in one sense, they had become as alike as identical twins."[7] The corn leaf blight sent researchers rushing to the gene banks in search of genetic material to breed new blight-resistant varieties.

Until recently, gene-banking was a haphazard business. Collections would be built up by an individual researcher at a seed company or a university, and often disappear when funds ran out or the researcher died. Storage methods were usually primitive; seeds must be stored at a proper temperature, protected from pests and disease, and periodically grown out. Consequently, much genetic material—often sample collections that had been gathered over a lifetime of field research—was lost. I have heard some scientists say that there has been as much genetic erosion in gene banks as in the outdoors.

Currently—in response to demand for material for genetic research and concern about loss of genetic material around the world—new genetic resource conservation centers are being established in many places and the storage technology is improving. Seeds are stored with temperature and humidity control, and sometimes deep-frozen. The embryo-freezing process developed primarily for agricultural animals is also employed for laboratory animals. The Jackson Laboratory at Bar Harbor, Maine, has for some years been preserving mouse germplasm (about 30 million mice are used annually for research in the United States) by freezing embryos in liquid nitrogen. Surrogate mother mice must then be used when the embryos are thawed and brought to life.[8] There has also been great improvement in the information storage and retrieval systems; where until quite recently it was sometimes difficult to know what material was stored where, the U.S. government has now developed a computerized germplasm resources network to serve as a national data bank.

Most genetic resource storage is in the developed nations but there are important gene banks in Nigeria, India, China, and several Latin American countries.[9] Such centers may specialize in native varieties, but more often than not their collections include material from other parts of the world as well. Some genetic resource conservation centers have no native plants at all. The world's largest collection of banana trees is located in La Lima, Honduras; all of its 850-odd varieties are from Asia, where the banana originated.

One of the most ambitious gene-banking projects in the world is the International Rice Germplasm Centre in the Philippines. Its collection currently holds about 67,000 Asian rice cultivars, over 2500 African varieties, and 1100 wild rices; its program for the immediate future is to collect samples of *all* the remaining varieties—the global total of cultivars of O. *sativa* and O. *glaberrima* is estimated at over 120,000—and to maintain for posterity the results of thousands of years of natural evolution and human selection.[10]

The word "resource" is often used now in connection with genetic material, and this is the key word in a new kind of political controversy that has arisen along with the increasing awareness of genetic erosion, the booming international seed industry, and the rapidly-developing science and technology of germplasm conservation.

The world's political leaders are beginning to understand that genetic material is a resource—a resource, furthermore, that comes from the less developed nations but is chiefly controlled by the developed ones. The United States is indeed one of the world's great food-producing nations, but the genetic information that supports American agriculture comes from other places. New genetic information is regularly introduced into the standard crop varieties— "topping off," the seed people call it—to improve them and protect them against new diseases. It is an ongoing evolutionary race, pests and diseases against crops. The scientists from the developed nations make their regular treks to distant regions to gather seeds and cuttings, and some people now ask whether a royalty or restitution is not owed to the nations from which the genetic material is taken. This genetic material, found in the Vavilov centers and similar regions, becomes more valuable with the advent of genetic technology. Until recently, the seed industry has had only a limited ability to make use of exotic distant relatives of the major crops plants, but that situation will change dramatically as it becomes possible to splice genes directly.

Representatives of the developed nations say genetic material is "the common heritage of mankind" and should be freely available to scientists and farmers everywhere. Mooney and other critics of the seed industry counter that the "common heritage" position is seriously weakened when the seed companies patent plants and then sell them to Third World farmers. There are other restrictions on the free exchange of genetic material. The seed storage bank at Fort Collins (the world's largest storehouse of genetic material) regularly sends seeds to foreign scientists on request—but has been known to refuse material to some nations for what the U.S. Department of Agriculture called "political reasons." Among the nations that have been refused material are the Soviet Union, Cuba, Iran, Libya, and Nicaragua.[11]

Many countries have laws against exporting germplasm of their major cash crops: Ecuador guards the secret of its cocoa, Ethiopia its wild coffee trees, Iraq its date palm, and I have heard reports of capital punishment for smuggling wild pistachio nuts out of Iran. These prohibitions, however, work about as well as most such governmental efforts—i.e., not very—and germplasm of all kinds is freely exchanged among scientists around the world.

At meetings of the United Nations' Food and Agriculture Organization in the early 1980s, control of genetic resources became an international issue. The lines in the controversy were drawn between the developed nations and the Third World. Mexico, taking a leadership role among the Third World nations, proposed an international gene bank and a legal agreement among member nations to insure the full exchange of plant genetic materials. The proposals became the subject of heated, often angry, debate, with the United States the leading opponent and virtually all Third World nations—including the closest of U.S. allies, even El Salvador—supporting them.

At the 1983 meeting of the FAO, delegates adopted a compromise version of the free-exchange agreement—a voluntary "undertaking" that the countries are not required to sign or live by—and preliminary steps toward the establishment of an international gene bank.

For the delegates to the FAO and the governments they represent, the issue is chiefly one of control, and closely resembles the Law of the Seas debate over ocean resources. Mooney's book about it is aptly entitled *The Law of the*

Seed. It is an issue linked to other conflicts between the developed and developing nations, and it has to do with the most basic of all human resources—the seeds that make it possible to produce food and fiber from the soil. Third World leaders speak of opportunities to maintain control of their genetic resources and develop agriculture suited to their peoples' needs. The American officials who represented the Reagan administration during the controversy see the conflict as a hypocritical attempt by the Third World countries (many of which prohibit exchange of seeds of their own cash crops) to get the high-grade seeds which are the stock in trade of the seed companies.

It is a game of international biopolitics played out against the backdrop of a rapidly changing world and informed by a rapidly changing genetic science. Once the Vavilov Centers were the repositories of genetic variety, now the seed banks are taking that role. While the technology of seed storage is improving, some scientists are working on a more sophisticated technology: storage of genes instead of seeds, "gene libraries" instead of seed banks. Beyond that is the possibility of yet another level: storage of formulas instead of genes, data banks instead of gene libraries, with the genes being created mechanically upon demand. In that technology, genetic information would literally become symbolic information.

The latter development is far beyond present capabilities, and more in the territory of science fiction than public policy. But there is an important political issue connected with such ideas. Genetic resource people tend to divide into two camps: those who want to preserve material *in situ,* that is in its natural habitat—in protected areas, or in farms that are operated as living seed banks; and those who want to preserve it *ex situ,* in seed banks, or arboreta or zoos or "gene libraries" not vulnerable to the many dangers it is subject to in the field. This is a controversy that may in time turn into a more cooperative venture as people recognize that, given the pressures, all kinds of gene banking operations are needed.

But the germplasm cannot be stored in any form if it is lost for all time, and that is what is now happening to much of it. For many people who are involved in this field the overwhelming concern is not who controls the material or how it is stored, but whether it is saved at all. One biologist said to me early in 1984: "If the work is not done in the next five to ten years, we're finished."

Patenting Life

ONE OF the most critical issues in evolutionary governance—likely to be a subject of controversy for decades if not centuries to come—is patenting. Although the practice of protecting the intellectual "property" of inventors and artisans dates back to the Middle Ages, patenting is essentially a child of the Industrial Revolution—one that is taking on a whole new life in the early years of the Biological Revolution.

The social usefulness of patenting has always been debatable. The argument in favor of it rests on the justice of rewarding creative people and on the belief that the promise of patent-guaranteed profits spurs research and development. Opponents of patenting call it a state-protected monopoly, and point out that all patents rest on an evolution of research, and that quite often the person or corporation who takes out a patent has contributed very little to the "discovery" upon which it proceeds to amass great wealth.

The current controversy is about the patenting of living things—seeds, organisms. The boom in selective breeding of plants that followed on Mendel's work led to widespread demands for legal protection of what became known as Plant Breeders' Rights, PBR for short, and in 1930 the United States became the first country to respond with legislation. Before that time, all living organisms were legally in the public domain. The Plant Patent Act of 1930 allowed patenting of asexually propagated plants (those not normally grown from seed), thus making it possible for the creators of various new flowers, fruits, trees, and ornamental shrubs to profit from their work as from any non-living invention. Although the idea of plant patenting had strong international opposition, it gained great momentum among the plant-breeding European nations. In the 1960s the International Union for the Protection of New Plant Varieties was founded; several countries enacted laws that went farther than the American model and extended patent protection to seeds. The United States caught up in 1970 with the Plant Variety Protection Act, which enlarged the scope of protection to include sexually reproducing plants as well.[12] This law had been proposed by the American Seed Trade Association; it was opposed by consumers, farmers, scientists, and large wholesale users of farm products such as the Campbell Soup Company. Campbell and other major purchasers of vegetable stocks were concerned about the likely price rises that would result, and the law was changed to exempt the soup vegetables—tomatoes, peppers, cucumbers, okra, carrots, and celery.[13] But the seed companies ultimately prevailed, and these vegetables also were given protection under amendments passed in 1980.

So in a fairly short period of time, with almost no awareness on the part of the general public, a massive legal transition has taken place: There is now a global system of plant-patenting laws and, nested within it, a seed industry that is one of the world's fastest-growing fields of research, development, and commerce. Genetic information is now patentable, at least in the plant kingdom, and there is much talk of extending similar protection to new animal varieties; the American Bar Association, not surprisingly, is strongly in favor of it. Whatever may be the impact of patenting on the global gene pool, it is definitely good news for lawyers.

The question of the evolutionary consequences of the sudden emergence of a global system of plant patenting laws is not easily answered. One side claims that patenting increases genetic diversity, another that it reduces it.

The pro-patent group points to the undeniable increase in the number of varieties of certain kinds of crop plants, such as the numerous new kinds of wheat developed after passage of the 1970 law. The other side argues that much of the development of new varieties does not result from patent protection, but from other conditions—such as the development of a jet-propelled global food trade that stimulates winter crops of cereals and growing seasons of two or three crops a year, and the development of computer technology for keeping track of crossbreeding. Shell, one of the transnational plant-breeding giants, can now keep track of more than a million individual plants this way.[14] The opponents of patenting also point out that there is sometimes not much variety in the varieties: When the corn blight struck in the United States in 1970, it proved equally destructive to several brands of corn which had different trademarks but similar genes. And, finally, there is no doubt that many different local varieties or landraces are disappearing. The overall trend is toward more new human-created and patented varieties—their parents the seed companies and their home the gene banks—with fewer varieties created by natural selection or small farmers and surviving in the regions of natural genetic diversity.

Biotech: Whose Cornucopia?

THE ISSUES connected with genetic erosion link closely to those connected with biotechnology. For one thing, the new genetic technologies provide further evidence of the value—and the vulnerability—of the world's genetic resources. Gene-splicing, cell fusion, tissue culture and the other developing methods of high-tech evolution are basically new ways of working with the genetic information that already exists in the world. Although some research is based on synthesized material, the new technologies chiefly draw on the genetic library that evolution had assembled before the human species knew how to read its information. The Biological Revolution spectacularly increases human capability to make use of genetic information—at the same time that the global supply of such information is rapidly diminishing.

The news about the new genetic technologies has been so dominated by gene-splicing, and by a single policy issue connected with it—the potential for massive biological disaster—that relatively little attention has been paid to the control and priority issues: what is produced first, for whom and by whom; who decides what is produced; and who decides who decides. That is to say, relatively little attention has been paid by the general public and its tribunes in the mass media. Much attention has been paid by specialists and interest groups, and a system of decision-making is well established. Its main components are research and development funding, and patent protection.

R & D priorities are not allocated on the basis of debate and public dialogue. Sometimes they express a broad-based and unquestioned social consensus, as did the massive interest in space research that followed the launching of the Sputnik satellite by the Soviet Union in the 1950s or the costly and much-publicized "war on cancer" of the 1970s. Public funding of cancer research was one of the forces that brought the new genetic technologies into being, and it is one of the main reasons why gene-splicing has produced medical results more rapidly than agricultural ones; there is no comparable base of agricultural research for the genetic industry to build upon.

Although the U.S. government and other national governments have been major sources of R & D funding, some of the large foundations are centers of R & D power that easily rival governments; a reasonable case could be made that the Rockefeller Foundation has made as many major decisions in evolutionary governance as any federal agency. It was midwife and nursing mother to the science of molecular biology (so named by a foundation official)[15] and its support of that science came far in advance of the massive public funding that began when the U. S. government launched its war on cancer. The Rockefeller Foundation was also the backer of the Green Revolution and the sponsor of CIMMYT, the rice- and wheat-research center and gene bank in Mexico. Foundations make their decisions in private and are not answerable to the public, but those decisions generally represent a vision of the public interest and often shape the course of public policy. The Green Revolution, for example, was one of the most important things that has been done by the developed nations to direct the course of agricultural development in the Third World.

Allocation of R & D money by private corporations often builds on earlier research—a matter of constant irritation to critics on the Left who see the corporations ripping off the profits from publicly-funded science—and is aimed at specific targets. At least, corporate officials *try* to aim funding at specific targets; in practice, the early years of the marriage between biotechnology and business were rocky ones, with corporations having great difficulty at targeting funding and producing the results desired by venture capitalists. Burke Zimmerman says in his study of the biotechnology business: "The concept of 'directed' research, except to solve a very well-defined practical problem, is continually proved wrong. The most useful discoveries often come from where one least expects to find them." [16]

The whole structure of corporate R & D financing in biotechnology is connected to patenting. Without the possibility of obtaining a legal patent on a process—or, as is now possible, a life form—the incentives and costs would be much different.

There was a good deal of publicity about the *Chakrabarty v. Diamond* decision which made legal history by allowing a human being to take out a patent on an organism created through recombinant DNA technology: man patents microbe. Novel as this was, it represented—like other aspects of biotechnology—a step along a general line of development rather than an entirely new departure. The *Chakrabarty* patent would never have been granted if the American Seed Association had not paved the way by lobbying the plant patent acts of 1930 and 1970 into existence; these were the laws that were cited before the Court (by both sides, since there were different possible interpretations of what the United States Congress had had in its august mind when it passed them), and were the basis of the decision.

The research that led to the decision was the work of a scientist named Ananda M. Chakrabarty, an employee of General Electric, who had "invented" a microorganism that ate crude oil, digesting it into harmless byproducts. The commercial agenda which had brought this small life form into being was the possibility of its use to clean up oil spills. Three separate patent claims were involved in the *Chakrabarty* case: one for the process whereby the oil-eating bacterium was created, one for the bacterium itself, and one for a product made up of bacteria and the straw that kept it floating on water. The Patent Office allowed the claims on the process and the product, but rejected the claim on the bacterium itself. General Electric brought suit on behalf of Chakrabarty and the Court decided that the bacterium qualified as a "composition of matter" and was patentable. The majority held that, in permitting the patenting of plants, Congress had recognized that the "relevant distinction was not between living and inanimate things, but between products of nature, whether living or not, and man-made organisms."[17]

That was one breakthrough: Protein engineering promises still more, as companies seek protection for "muteins".

Diversifying Genetic Technology

THE PATENT laws—and the court interpretations that extend them to biotechnology—are part of the institutional structure that determines where the power in the Biological

Revolution resides. In the United States, priority-allocating power over the new biotechnologies rests firmly in the private sector. The federal government has provided funding for basic research, but has not volunteered any answers to the questions that the late political scienctist Harold Lasswell declared to be the very essence of politics—namely who gets what, when, how. The Reagan administration quashed a few feeble attempts by White House staff members to define public interest or mediate among private interests in regard to the emerging technologies, and did not choose to launch any scientific crusades on the model of the space program or the war on cancer that might have pointed them in any particular direction. In the absence of such guidance, priority-allocating decisions have chiefly been market decisions.

This is not necessarily good or bad in itself, but it is of profound importance to many people. Some of the new biochemicals produced through recombinant DNA technology can greatly improve the quality of life for certain people. Often—not neccessarily always—"zero sum" choices are made. Had the industry not moved quickly into producing human insulin, some of those same economic and scientific resources might have been allocated toward the production of some other biochemical that would make life better for some other group of people. Such a choice would not have been an absolute one: Sooner or later science will probably explore all the possibilities and the biotech industries will market every product for which there is a buyer—but the "sooner or later" means a great deal. If you were a parent whose child had been born a congenital dwarf, you would feel strongly about whether growth hormone became available now or five or ten years from now.

Also, diseases tend to afflict people of certain races, regions, age groups or social classes. Diabetes has such a demographic preference, which appears to result from both genetic and environmental causes. As a British writer puts it, "Most diabetics are made by their diet, even if potential diabetics are born."[18] The diet is the high-fat, high-sugar, low-fibre food consumed by people in the developed countries; diabetes is one of the group sometime called "Western Diseases."[19] More specifically, it is primarily to be found among people of advanced years in Western countries. This is a good market. But some people argue, citing persuasive medical evidence, that there would be much greater health payoffs—fewer diabetics—if people in the Western world ate differently. Others are concerned that a decision has been made to produce yet another product for a Western disease instead of directing attention to one of the many tropical diseases that kill or maim thousands of people and for which modern science has produced no cure or preventive vaccine.

According to the World Health Organization, one category of disease—the enteric diseases—is the cause of 80 percent of illness worldwide. This classification includes cholera, typhoid fever, and the bacterial and amoebic dysenteries. These are estimated to cause 20 million deaths annually. Second in importance are the parasitic diseases like malaria, filiariasis, and river blindness. All of these diseases are more common in the Third World than in the developed nations, are major scourges of humanity, and have been regularly undervalued as investment priorities by the leading pharmaceutical firms although promising avenues of research have been opened up by the new biotechnologies.[20]

Similar issues arise in regard to agricultural priorities. For example, will biotechnology make farmers less dependent on chemicals, or moreso? One biotechnology entrepreneur, David Padwa, says that "In time, the entire insecticide industry may be totally displaced by plant genetics."[21] But some American biotech companies are excited about the possibility of producing plants that will be resistant to herbicide or other agricultural chemicals, thereby making it possible for farmers to use those potions *more* liberally than they could otherwise. In fact, several companies that manufacture agricultural chemicals are among the major supporters of agricultural biotechnology. Obviously, new crops whose growth is linked to heavy chemical use are going to be of greater appeal to practitioners of Western-style mechanized agribusiness than to Third World peasants who are hard put to afford such chemicals in any quantity.

There are also potential environmental and health impacts involved in increased *chemical* use: impacts that are a matter of public interest. The U.S. federal and state governments have environmental protection agencies that, with varying degrees of effectiveness, represent this public interest; most foreign countries have no such mechanism. One of the global environmental disasters of our time is the widespread and often incredibly heavy use of American-made agricultural chemicals that have been banned in the U.S. As of this writing new moves are underway to deal with that problem—both by placing new import restrictions on American-made chemicals, and by creating better regulatory systems in the countries where they are used. Meanwhile, in California, the newspapers report on a growing volume of lawsuits against manufacturers and users of agricultural chemicals: Suits alleging birth defects, cancer and other chronic health effects as a result of exposure to toxic chemicals are clogging the courts and providing a new growth industry for lawyers.[22] I mention these developments—not directly concerned with genetic technology—because they point out one way that the public sector can influence what biotechnology does. Any country (or state) with a body of strong toxic chemical legislation and an informed and vigilant public ready to sue polluters is a place in which the private sector decision-makers will think hard about ways to reduce the use of toxic chemicals. Some kinds of biotechnological products can do this, and others cannot.

Jack Doyle of the Environmental Policy Institute in Washington, D.C., sees a potential for a biotechnological "soft path," in which the new science would focus on such products as genetically engineered viruses or bacteria that would kill insects, or crops genetically engineered to resist disease or pests without the use of chemicals. Several companies are doing research in this direction and a couple are close to being ready to market biological pesticides. But this does not add up to a stampede down the soft path. One research executive says that neither the chemical industry nor state and federal governments are concerned enough about the undesirable side effects of chemical insecticides to give top priority to exploring the vast range of new nonchemical alternatives that genetic technology opens up.[23]

There has been much talk about how the new biotechnologies might be harnessed to the service of interests other than Western industry, Western medicine and Western agribusiness—much talk, but little action. One project that may amount to something—and which is strikingly parallel in its political alignments to the controversy over control of genetic resources—is the move to establish a world center for biotechnology.

The idea of an International Center for Genetic Engineering and Biotechnology, as it came to be called in the early 1980s, sprang from the widely-held belief that (a) genetic engineering could do great things for the developing nations, and (b) left to its own devices, it would probably do great things for the developed nations first. The benefits of (a) were being somewhat oversold at the time by news stories that indicated great medical and agricultural breakthroughs just around the corner, but there was no doubt that the Third World stood to be left as far behind the Biological Revolution as it had been by the Industrial.

The idea was not to attempt to compete with or influence the Western biotechnology industry, but to set up, under United Nations auspices, a research center to look for ways the new science and technology might be of value to the Third World. There were many mistakes made in the early stages of this project and a lot of the political in-fighting that regularly arises among Third World nations when they decide to unite on something. Diplomats intrigued over such issues as where the proposed center should be located. Scientific consultants believed the center should be located in a Western nation where it might be close to major universities and assured of trained technical personnel and adequate supplies and equipment; most delegates favored locating it in a Third World nation. It was finally decided, in a decision that may prove more politic than practical, to establish two sites: one in Europe, one in India.

It is too early to say how successful the international center will prove to be, but the main political forces in regard to control and priority-setting in biotechnology are clearly evident. One force, easily the more powerful, is the market force represented by the biotechnology industry; the other is the collectivist force represented by the international center. This does not necessarily imply conflict so much as diversity—an attempt to set up an institution empowered to act according to different priorities and different values than those which drive the biotech companies. The founders of the international center clearly recognize where the expertise is, and hope to draw on it in their own activities.

Enlightened policy on the part of the Western nations would be to encourage both sides: to foster conditions of free research and healthy competition in the industry, and to give some aid and support to the international center. Very few have done so, and the U.S. was one of the least supportive of the international center. The Reagan administration refused to contribute material aid to the center, boycotted planning meetings held by the sponsoring agency (the United Nations Industrial Development Organization), and even forbade the U.S. Embassy in Belgrade to send an observer to the first organizing coference held there.[24]

The American press paid no attention to any of this, any more than it had to U.S. seed policy as expressed at the FAO conference in Rome. No newspaper editorials questioned American policy in regard to global priorities for biotechnology, no presidential candidate criticized the Reagan administration policy in the 1984 campaign. As far as the public and the mass media were concerned, the only policy issue connected to biotechnology was whether the scientists should be prevented from manufacturing a genetic Frankenstein.

Another Modern Prometheus?

MEDIA REPORTS about biotechnology have tended to concentrate on recombinant DNA, and have oscillated between hype and hysteria: between overstatements of the wonders likely to accrue from genetic engineering—the "pork chops on trees" school of reportage—and fearsome speculations about the possible dangers.

The scientific community has tried to cool down the rhetoric and keep its hand on the gavel, without much success; it has been torn by its own ambivalence between great hopes and great fears, and some of its attempts to assess the risks of research have fed rather than allayed public concern. In the mid-1970s, poised on the brink of the Biological Revolution, genetic scientists took the unprecedented action of accepting a moratorium on recombinant DNA experimentation until general safety guidelines could be adopted, and held an historic conference at Asilomar, California, to discuss the implications of their work.

They did so expecting that these actions would reassure the public. Instead they prompted a wave of articles about the hazards of recombinant DNA research.

The basic problem was that recombinant DNA experiments using *E. coli* bacteria were being performed by biochemists and molecular biologists, rather than by microbiologists who were accustomed to doing animal cell culture work and to taking the necessary steps required to maintain laboratory sterility.[25] This might produce a disease-causing strain of bacteria and some accident might allow it to infect lab workers or the public. Some scientists suggested ways that experiments might generate cancer-producing DNA, or substances that could disturb human biochemical functioning. These were frightening scenarios, but nothing compared to those that began to appear in the media.

The public and the press did not yet know much about recombinant DNA technology, but everybody had seen a monster movie or two and the discussion soon escalated to talk of global epidemics and high-tech Frankensteins. When the city council of Cambridge, Massachusetts was deliberating about adopting its own set of guidelines to govern research at Harvard and MIT, Mayor Alfred Vellucci made a speech about seven-foot-tall monsters emerging from the Boston sewers.[26] He got a lot of headlines. The *New York Times Magazine* ran an article entitled "New Strains of Life—or Death," which warned of the possibility that a laboratory technician might pour a cancer-causing germ culture down a sink drain, where the bacteria would transfer their malignant properties to other bacteria which would be discharged into the ocean near shellfish beds, and that people eating the shellfish would then get infectious cancer which might spread in epidemic proportions.[27]

Public discussions had a tendency to bring out science-fiction images that had nothing to do with the safety of *E. coli* experiments. At a 1977 forum held by the National Academy of Sciences to promote public discussion of the issues connected with recombinant DNA research, followers of biotechnology opponent Jeremy Rifkin temporarily broke up the meeting while singing "We shall not be cloned," although cloning human beings was hardly the issue being discussed.[28] Many scientists, unaccustomed to such antics, began to wish they had never brought up the subject.

For a while it seemed that the matter was politically charged enough to make it worth some legislator's while to enact the guidelines into law, but after a few members of Congress moved in that direction the enterprise ran out of momentum.

There were several reasons why Congress did not take the unprecedented step of turning the guidelines—mandatory for scientists working under National Institute of Health grants, advisory for others—into federal law. One reason was that scientists lobbied against it, another was that lawmakers always have many things to do and that one got lost in the shuffle—but the chief reason was that there was little public support for such a move. Since the issue, once it got into the public arena, had been defined in terms of whether recombinant DNA experimentation might lead to plagues, monsters, and human clones, the only available choice seemed to be hysteria or apathy. Most people chose apathy, and one can hardly blame them.

Guidelines for safety in DNA research were adopted in the U.S. and several countries. The moratorium ended, and soon recombinant DNA work with *E. coli* bacteria was routine in research laboratories and universities everywhere. A few years ago a high school biology class in Denmark successfully completed a gene-splicing experiment.[29] Meanwhile, other researchers designed experiments to test the hazard scenarios: One built a model sewage treatment plant and ran a gene-spliced strain of *E. coli* through it to see if significant amounts of its marker plasmid transferred to other bacteria in sewage—which it did not.[30] The absence of any mishap over the first decade or so of widespread recombinant DNA research does not prove that the new biotechnologies are "safe"—only that certain kinds of work can be performed using safeguards that are roughly the same as those used in similar bacterial research. The absence of seven-foot monsters emerging from the Boston sewers proves that some of the issues raised by people scrambling for a role of political leadership in relation to biotechnology have no relevance whatever to the real issues, and serve to widen the gulf between the public and the scientific community—instead of narrowing it and helping to lay a foundation for informed participation in the politics of the Biological Revolution.

As research on agricultural applications of the new biotechnologies progresses, we have to deal with the possible risks involved in releasing genetically modified life forms into the environment. The public got a preview of this in the early 1980s when Rifkin brought suit to halt an experiment in which genetically altered bacteria would be used to retard frost damage on plants. Some bacteria enable ice crystals to form, but others, lacking a gene that facilitates that chemical process, do not. Two scientists at the University of California proposed to saturate a row of potato plants with the altered bacteria, thus filling up the econiche and enabling the potatoes to survive at lower temperatures. This is a piece of "soft path" biotechnology, since the common practice of farmers is to use pesticides to control the ice-forming bacteria. The researchers believed their experiment to be safe since ice-resistant bacteria exist in nature and have also been produced and disseminated artificially using "conventional" culture technology with no ill effects; also, the modified bacteria had had nothing added—only a gene deleted. Rifkin charged that the modified bacteria might multiply in large numbers and drastically alter the region's plant and insect population, perhaps spreading into the clouds where they would reduce snowfall and spring runoff.[31] The weather-modification scenario reared its head again in 1986 when another group was preparing to test "ice minus" bacteria in a strawberry field in Monterey County. Some environmental publications reprinted the scenario as if it were gospel: "By reducing the freezing level of rain falling over major mountain ranges," said *Earth Island Journal*, " 'Ice-Minus' could significantly reduce snowfall. Not only would ski resorts suffer the impact of reduced snowpacks but, even more troubling, increased runoff could trigger massive flooding of hills and lowlands."[32]

In such controversies, genetically engineered microorganisms are likened to exotic species. Tens of thousands of exotic species of plant and animal life have moved or been moved to other environments. Most have perished. Many—like the potatoes and strawberries that people wanted to test ice-minus bacteria on—can survive when cared for. A few of them cause major ecological damage; some favorite examples are the Asian fungus that virtually wiped out the American chestnut tree, the Japanese kudzu vine that blankets the American South, the European starlings that make life miserable for American farmers, the gypsy moths that munch through American trees. The question is whether the products of genetic technology are capable of getting out of hand in the same way. The scientists doing the research believe they are only minutely different from organisms already present in the environment. Other scientists feel less secure about this, and some people believe that genetic modification is per se an intervention of another order with a much greater potential of producing large-scale ecological disturbances.

The question can be stated in general terms, but it can only be answered by analyzing each case as it arises. Such an investigative and learning process is going to be the task of decades and probably centuries to come. It is going to require an immense amount of work, it is going to call for a lot of governmental regulation, and it is going to need a much better class of public dialogue than it has produced so far.

The public dialogue is debased not only by the lurid rhetoric of the Mayor Vellucci variety about what might result from biotechnology, but also by misleading statements of how society can control evolution. In another genetic-technology controversy that arose in the mid-1980s—this time about using growth hormone to produce larger varieties of sheep and pigs—Rifkin proposed that the government should "protect the biological integrity of every mammalian species." A biologist at Ohio University thought this was "a hilarious proposal," since it would legislate the right of all species to remain as they were and put the government in the position of decreeing a halt to even the natural process of evolution that is continually experimenting with all species.[33]

There may be good reasons for prohibiting the use of growth hormone for such purposes—but if we were to declare that the species boundary lines were legally uncrossable, we would have trouble from nature, where boundaries are rarely clear. Hybrids often appear, and have often been deliberately bred: mules, the hybrid pack camels of the Middle East, the Madura cattle of Indonesia, the "beefalo" now bred commercially in the United States. If Rifkin's proposal were adopted then there should be appropriate criminal punishment for creating a hybrid by crossbreeding. Some people who have done business with mules would not consider this an entirely bad idea, but we need to have some sense of scale about what kinds of constraints governments can impose—and people accept.

[130]

At other times other blanket prohibitions are proposed. Some advocate outlawing all genetic engineering involving animals and human beings. The West German Green party in 1986 passed a resolution opposing all industrial applications of biotechnology—presumably including toxic waste control. Frequently one hears of proposals to prohibit biotechnology altogether. The latter is a most simplistic reaction; it would require that genetic engineering be outlawed globally, and global society has so far failed to outlaw anything—even nuclear war, which might be a more reasonable thing to start with than a scientific revolution that is capable of producing real benefits along with perplexing problems. Another weakness in the idea is that such a ban would be unenforcable even if adopted, since DNA experimentation is relatively simple and inexpensive; to stamp it out would require a global police state that might be at least as vexing as frost-free potatoes and oversized pigs, and a kind of thought control that we have not seen since the days of the Inquisition.

A Special Moral Position

MARK LAPPÉ, a scientist and writer on public health policy, says that biotechnology "creates an unprecedented opportunity for benefiting humanity" and that the new industry should be accorded a "special moral position" in society.[34]

If there is any position the biotechnology industry's leaders would *not* like to occupy, a special moral one is it. They want biotechnology to be taken seriously, but not *too* seriously. If the world expects too much from it, its progress through the golden halls of venture capital is likely to be disturbed by demands that it pursue problems and projects that have little commercial appeal.

Malaria presents a case in point. It is, to begin with, one of humanity's leading health problems: It afflicts some 250 million people a year worldwide and kills a million people a year in Africa alone. It also presents a formidable technolgical challenge, since it produces a different antigen at each stage of the parasitic cycle and an effective vaccine would probably have to be a "cocktail" of three different antibodies.[35] Genetic technology appears capable of accomplishing this feat, but the industry has been reluctant to commit itself to malaria vaccine research. The vaccine is simply not a good commercial prospect: It would require a long and costly research effort before producing a saleable product, and the market would then be—as a Genentech executive put it—"ill-defined, diffuse, and dependent upon governmental sponsorship or advertising." Genentech, the company that developed genetically-engineered human insulin, had been asked by the World Health Organization to take part in developing a malaria vaccine prototype, and had declined. The project was not, as the same executive frankly stated, "compatible with Genentech's business strategy."[36] This decision is no doubt unassailable from a business point of view, but it illustrates dramatically why so many people believe a pure business point of view is not good enough in determining how biotechnology is to be used. Progress toward developing a malaria vaccine is being made, but only through efforts supported by public funds and foundation grants; if recombinant DNA technology conquers malaria, as I believe it will, the world will owe a great deal to biotechnology and nothing at all to the biotechnology industry.

Another point to be considered in regard to biotechnology's moral position is its potential for developing new methods of biological warfare. There is no doubt that this potential exists, and I believe that research on military applications is being carried out in both the United States and the Soviet Union. Use of any toxin or disease-creating agent is covered by existing treaties on biological warfare, but there are many ways that research can proceed: It can be overtly military with a "defensive" orientation, or it can be directed into subjects which can have *either* health or military applications. The loopholes are big enough that many researchers have been able to proceed with work under Defense Department contracts.

Lappé proposes a broadly based set of public and private actions to prevent biotechnology from turning its promise into new weaponry that might make the nuclear nightmare seem pleasant by comparison: among them, giving public health a clear priority in all recombinant DNA research, withholding federal funds from any research not directed to health or peace, and putting the public sector research community (i.e., the universities) off-limits as contractors for classified Department of Defense biological research.[37]

Biotechnology's special moral position is defined by its great capacity for doing good and its great capacity for doing evil. The more clearly these become publicly understood, the more people are likely to ask that its decisions be not simply matters of business strategy, but reflections of public—and global—interest. This is no reason to sell your biotechnology stock: The industry will undoubtedly market many products and create many millionaires. But it will do so with the world looking over its shoulder. Biotechnology has become an industry and will doubtless become a very important one—and yet it is not *only* an industry; it is a part of global evolution, and it is everybody's business.

No doubt the many opponents and critics of biotechnology will applaud the idea of its occupying such a public role. But if biotechnology is to be given a special moral position, then we are required to take a special moral position toward it as well. Biotechnology is capable of being exploited in many ways: It can be milked for profit, it can be mobilized for military power, and—because it is an emerging and attention-getting field of public policy— it can provide a sudden source of influence, fame, and other heady rewards for anyone who captures a mass-media role in opposition to it. Its appearance has generated some searching dialogue, some very bad journalism, and some outright demagoguery. Images of human clones and monsters have been regularly invoked in the press. Anti-biotech activists have dealt with the industry as though it were a malevolent legion of mad scientists, and have felt free to insert lurid scenarios of genetic disaster into every controversy as though by doing so they were raising the public consciousness.

The public deserves better. It is not going to be stampeded into evolutionary responsibility by repeated exposure to carelessly-concocted predictions of catastrophe. If anything, when such predictions regularly prove to be incorrect, people will only be more likely to fail to take the real dangers seriously, or to trouble themselves to learn about the difficult issues involved. There is no doubt that biotechnology is dangerous; manipulations of life systems are always dangerous. But we need to think clearly and be honest about those dangers. There are too many opportunities to distort them, and to create public hysteria. Much of the contemporary concern has the same dynamic as public fear of communism in the 1950s. It is true that there are revolutions that produce Marxist states; it is true that people sometimes do things that create huge biological messes. But not every popular movement is a communist conspiracy, and not every intervention is a massive ecological disaster. To suggest the latter, which has become the standard procedure of the Jeremy Rifkins of the world, is biological McCarthyism.

There is a lot to be learned, including the lesson of how to go about debating the issues. The question of field-testing genetically altered organisms is a particularly touchy one, and has given rise to an extensive interdisciplinary dialogue between molecular biologists and ecologists. The ecologists' concern is very much like that of microbiologists during the 1970s discussion of the safety of laboratory research. The microbiologists had been working with lethal organisms for decades, had developed a body of knowledge and safety procedures, and were concerned that the scientists working with recombinant DNA learn the appropriate microbiological techniques.[38] And the main reason DNA laboratory research proceeded to establish a good safety record was that biochemists and molecular biologists did learn and apply that kind of knowledge. Similarly, in the more recent dialogue, the outcome has to be closer collaboration between somewhat overspecialized separate disciplines—in this case, molecular biologists and ecologists. As an ecologist put it during a scientific conference about engineered organisms in the environment: "If genetic engineering is the cutting edge, then maybe ecology is the whetstone."[39]

These are not merely arcane matters to be deliberated at scientific conferences. The possibility of ecological disturbance from use of genetically altered organisms demands good science, strict regulation by agencies of government, and an informed and skeptical public. Biotechnology is a moral concern, and the debate about its hazards must be a public one. It follows that whoever enters into the debate has an obligation to try to produce a high quality of public dialogue—ecologicaly informed, prudent, and striving to get at the truth. We cannot rely on the "self-policing" of the biotechnology industry, and the public should be vigilant and critical of the industry and of its proposals. We should also be vigilant and critical of those who offer themselves as our protectors, and should demand better reportage on biotechnology-related issues than the media have so far provided.

Biological Border Patrols

THE FOURTH component of the genetic rapids—the global travel of plant and animal life—is the one least noticed, although isolated cases occasionally make the headlines. One such case, the infestation of Mediterranean fruit flies in California in the early 1980s, was a major reason why then-governor Edmund G. Brown, Jr., later lost the election for the United States Senate. It was a highly technical issue with undercurrents of machismo and warfare. The state had been invaded from without, and a powerful interest group—agriculture—thought that the governor had been insufficiently forceful in repelling the foreigners.

The governor was, without quite knowing it, caught in a crunch of biopolitics; he was required to act as biological policeman, to intervene with force in the struggle for survival of non-human life forms—to exercise one of the most common but least-understood forms of political power, one that can cause trouble not only for governors but for nations and international organizations.

The migration of plant and animal life reflects the migration of human populations that has been the cause of many political conflicts. The nation-state, the predominant political organization of the modern era, rests on a concept of biological stability. The word "nation" implies a people of identifiable genetic homogeneity, a nationality; the word "state", closely akin to *static*, reflects the hope of keeping said people in control of a given piece of real estate. So through the eye of a true nationalist—Charles de Gaulle comes to mind—the world is ideally a place of neatly fenced-off fatherlands, each sovereign and distinct, each containing a population with its own recognizeable genetic and cultural identity.

Very few nation-states have ever measured up to the nationalist dream. There is a lot of truth in the old saying that a nation is a group of people united by a common error about their ancestry and a common dislike of their neighbors. Most nations contain large minorities of other nationalities—sometimes along their borders, sometimes in troublesome isolated pockets well within their sovereign territory. This has provided national governments with many occasions for doing the thing they do best, which is making war.

We now face similar problems about nonhuman immigrants. We have already noted that human migration is always ecosystem modification. The scale of such modifications increased greatly during the centuries of global exploration and empire-building: As European populations were established in the New World, edible plants and exotic pets were brought back to Europe, and ranches and plantations were carved out of the wilderness to serve a rapidly-growing international food trade. The scale is increasing again in our era of jet travel, mass migrations, frozen embryos, and seed banks.

There have been many political controversies about human migration and a general recognition of need for public policy to regulate it, but relatively little sustained interest in the movement of plants and animals and the ecosystem modification that results from it. This neglect is consistent with the human tendency to underestimate the extent of interventions, and reflects the scarcity of ecological thinking in political ideologies. On the whole, governments have supported programs to import exotic life forms that might be usable, and have aided farmers and ranchers in their efforts to stamp out native predators or weeds that do not get along with herds or crops—policies clearly favoring exotics when they are commercially valuable. A Western rancher may be xenophobic about a lot of things, but he will side with a foreign-bred cow against an American coyote any day of the week. The federal and state governments have also imported exotic game animals and stocked rivers with foreign fish for the pleasure of American sportsmen. On the whole, national governments have regarded the transplantation of life forms from one ecosystem to another as natural and good, but currently they are being forced to confront a surprisingly large number of exceptions to the rule.

One problem is the trade in rare or endangered species. Unfortunately, the more rare a species becomes, the higher the price for a specimen of it and the more interesting it is to collectors.

While zoos are undoubtedly part of the solution in the human effort to preserve endangered species, they are also a part of the problem: Zookeepers frequently purchase animals that have been illegally captured, and even more frequently look away from the brutal and wasteful methods employed in capture and shipment. Capturing wild animals often hastens extinction by disrupting breeding groups, and many animals die before reaching their destinations.

Far greater numbers of animals and plants go to private collectors. There is a huge international trade in tropical fish, and an equally huge one in exotic birds. Much of the latter is illegal also, and is the bizarre profession of a new breed of daring smugglers who board jet airliners with dozens of narcotized birds sewed into hidden pockets in their clothes. Many of the birds do not survive such travel, of course, but those that do command prices which make the effort worthwhile. The trade also includes monkeys, wild cats, snakes, lizards, tree frogs, and various other unlikely house pets—some of which are transported in large numbers, and few of which are really suitable for domestication. The International Union for the Conservation of Nature reported that, between 1967 and 1972, the United Kingdom imported 1.2 million specimens of a popular species of Moroccan tortoise, and estimated that 80 percent of them died in the first year of captivity.[40]

The direction of such trade is mainly South to North, from Third World to developed nations, but officials in the United States are also worried about the plunder of American wildlife. Some hunters search for a certain product—gall bladders from bears for sale as aphrodisiacs in Asian apothecary shops, eagle feathers to be made into Indian headdresses in France—while others capture animals and export them live: Hawks from Montana are fancied for use in falconry by Saudi Arabian royalty, and real American falcons have brought as much as $50,000 apiece from foreign connoisseurs.[41]

Cacti from the Southwest are another big international commodity. Some of this is legal trade and a sizeable one at that—around 10 million cacti a year are exported annually from Texas alone—and some of it is what Southwesterners call "cactus rustling": poaching from national parks, or collecting any of the seventy-odd species or varieties that are on the endangered list. The most spectacular recorded incident of cactus gathering took place when a group of Japanese merchants directed the removal of *all* the cacti from an island off the coast of Baja California.[42]

The movements of insect pests are the most destructive of such practices, and the hardest to control. California's adventure with the Mediterranean fruit fly is a classic example of the problems involved in policing an artificial ecosystem. For many years the state has had an elaborate border-control system to protect its citrus crops, but still there are the harbors and the airports, bringing people and products in from all over the world. And there are also the fruit trees, the very treasure the government was striving to protect: California, with a climate temptingly similar to that of the Mediterranean, had become home for all the trees that grow in the Mediterranean region; the fruit flies felt right at home here, even though they seemed like invaders to the orchard owners.

The first Mediterranean fruit fly was discovered in California in the summer of 1980, and a huge biopolitical controversy ensued. Farmers wanted the Medfly stamped out, eradicated. Once that would have been no problem, but the Santa Clara Valley, where the Medfly was discovered, had turned into one of the country's fastest-growing urban areas. Its residents, who had been reading in the papers about the chemical contamination of the Love Canal region in New York state and the radiation leakage from the Three Mile Island power plant in Pennsylvania, were unenthusiastic about having helicopters flying over at night to spray the valley with malathion.

Finally, after several different control methods had been tried, with California growers claiming to have lost millions of dollars in revenue because out-of-state buyers were reluctant to purchase California fruits, the state government went ahead and sprayed with malathion. That cost upwards of $70 million, not counting lawsuits from people who claimed their property or their health or their car's paint jobs had been damaged by the insecticide. The infestation ended—at least for the time being, but none of the parties to the dispute were left particularly happy with its outcome. The farmers thought the governor had waited too long to take strong action, and the urban environmentalists thought he had finally sold them out.

The Medfly case illustrates a couple of biopolitical realities: Protecting an artificial environment from invaders takes either great ingenuity and effort, or much money and brute force. And sometimes, when people in the same geographic area want the government to maintain different kinds of artificial environments—such as fruit orchards and sprawling suburbs—the government ends up having to make an unpopular decision.

Genetic Policy-Making: Governance on the Move

IN ORDER to think about economic policy you have to have an image of an economy: a whole system of transactions among banks and governments and corporations and individuals. You may do micro-economics and look at a small part, but the idea of the larger system is still essential; without it there is no basis for analysis or even for productive disagreement.

The same is true for evolutionary policy. We know about some of the parts, but we lack an idea of the whole. I offer the material in this chapter and the one before it as a preliminary step toward forming such an idea.

As we look at this material, certain trends become evident. We see a great amount of genetic change taking place, many things in motion. We can see something that was not true of other evolutionary upheavals, which is that one species is the central active agent. These observations yield a couple of useful general guidelines for thinking about evolutionary politics:

One: We have to learn how to think about something that is in motion. The person who seeks to keep things as they are is going to end up on the losing side, regardless of the purity of his or her motives. Agendas based on homeostasis—such as the idea of a steady-state economy— have doubtful prospects in a biologically turbulent world. Such a world is unlikely to permit social, political, or economic stability, and those who would build policies or ideologies for the times ahead had better learn to build on the run.

Two: More things move from the realm of nature to the realm of politics. As human power in nature grows, so do human interconnections. Anything done in one place has an impact somewhere else. Politics is made of such connections, especially when there is uncertainty about what the impacts will be; there is quantitatively more politics. This means that, just as it is going to be difficult to maintain stability, it is also going to be difficult to have "less government," as is the fond hope of conservatives and libertarians, and the person who yearns to be apolitical is quite out of luck.

A biologically-informed image of what is happening in the world challenges many of our traditional ideas about politics—yet we have to talk of the issues in the language we all know, even as we recognize that we are dealing with an obsolescent framework of thought. We still speak of the politics of who gets what, when, how.

Who gets what, when, how: In regard to the extinction of wild species, if present trends proceed on track, the issue is who does *not* get what in the future. A world depleted of wild species will have deprivations for people of all persuasions. The human race will get to find out what it is like to live in a world that is vastly different from the one we know today. And we will have reduced the options of future human evolution. As Peter Raven, one of the nation's leading botanists, puts it: "The entire basis of our civilization rests on a few hundred species out of the millions that might have been selected, and we have hardly begun to explore the properties of the remainder."[43] Future-oriented considerations remind us that even our most enlightened political systems have no built-in protections for the interests of future generations.

Yet it does not take unselfish concern for posterity to understand the value of maintaining a richness of life forms in the world. It makes sense in so many ways that the neat itemizations of the reasons for doing so often seem to be heaping words on something that most people comprehend already.

For whatever reasons, many people have been moved to act. The outlines of a global policy are visible: It includes national parks and wildlife preserves, zoos, laws to regulate hunting and exportation of endangered species, national policies such as those embodied in the U. S. Endangered Species Act, and local and private projects such as regional preserves and dedicated private land.[44] It requires bureaucracies and laws, but it can never be done by government alone, any more than governments can by fiat create economic prosperity. It takes a generally-held sense of the value of genetic diversity. And we may as well stand reminded that this whole enterprise is having a very small impact on the rate of extinction, and furthermore that even if the issue suddenly jumped to the top of our list of political priorities, thousands of species would still be lost. We are in no danger of establishing an evolutionary status quo. The task at hand is to keep options open and act in a way that is consistent with the knowledge of living in a world where extinction does not happen, but is caused.

Policy in this area will evolve rapidly. We are just beginning to get used to the idea of any kind of public policy to protect endangered species, and we will soon realize that any effort to protect species is in fact a form of ecosystem management: You cannot preserve any species without having some effect on the plants and animals with which it interacts. And different management approaches are also likely to have different evolutionary consequences. We know this is so when species are harvested or hunted: Trophy hunting, for example, removes large-antlered deer from the phenotype and results in a "selection" of small-antlered animals. The science of ecology is in its infancy, as is the field of public policy concerned with the protection of species and ecosystems. The two will develop together—under much pressure—and we will soon see a global politics of ecosystem management, with constant monitoring of endangered species and undoubtedly lots of arguments about what should be protected and how.

These same observations apply to genetic resources, but here we are dealing with a situation that is a more clear and direct consequence of human intervention: Many of the varieties now being lost were created by selective breeding. Also, since the plants and animals in question are the ones that produce our food and fiber, it is much easier to think of them as "resources"—a designation that troubles some lovers of wildlife. Utilitarian values readily apply, and so do the political questions that we might ask about any other resource: Who controls it? For whose benefit is it being used? Some countries are taking stock of their resources and gene banks are becoming more numerous, but on the whole genetic resources are not a high governmental priority and have not received public attention commensurate to their importance to our lives. Personally, I am not impressed by the arguments in favor of seed patenting, but I would be more willing to live with it if it were the product of public debate rather than the result of mediation between seed companies and soupmakers.

The new biotechnologies are not going to be outlawed, but they are going to be regulated. Research under federal funding is already subject to the National Institute of Health guidelines, and a much larger regulatory system is being created to deal with the testing of medical products and the assessment of environmental hazards: a "Coordinated Framework for Regulation of Biotechnoloy" which parcels out various responsibilities among the Food and Drug Administration, the Department of Agriculture, the Environmental Protection Agency, and the Occupational Safety and Health Administration. Many states have similar studies underway to determine what agency gets which piece of the biotechnological action.[45]

A regulatory framework, however brilliantly constructed, is not a policy, however. Policy requires allocation of priorities—and this is a matter that calls for public involvement, discussion of moral issues, and the asking of hard political questions. We are going to have to find ways to define social priorities in biotechnology and carry them out. I have heard many proposals for this: Barry Commoner says we should nationalize the whole industry.[46] Other people propose various public/private structures to conduct research and even manufacture items that might be neglected by the private sector. There are many possibilities, and sorting them out will be a central part of the politics of the decades just ahead.

The fourth part of the picture, the movement of plants and animals around the world, calls for other laws and regulations—and better enforcement of existing ones—to impede movements that are ecologically destructive or that contribute to species extinction. But it also needs a much greater general comprehension of how much movement has taken place already, and of how much of the familiar environment is the result of earlier immigrations. If this is understood, and if people know that such movement can never be entirely contained and that no methods of pest control are infallible, we will be better equipped to live in the ever-changing and hazardous world we have helped to create.

If evolutionary politics is to be informed by the *kubernetes* principle I described in the foregoing chapter, we will need a constant triangular interplay among scientists, the public and government—and ways of making that interplay more productive. The methodology of forecasting and assessing environmental impacts is going to have to be constantly reexamined. The National Environmental Protection Act was a great innovation in its time, but it needs to be strengthened and improved. So does the public perception of what environmental impact statements are and do. Frequently they are viewed as scientific findings— which they are not—that tell just what is going to happen when a project is completed—which they cannot do. One recent study proposed that impact statements could come to be used as true scientific hypothethes about how the environment would be affected by a particular project. The project would then become a public ecological experiment, with extensive monitoring of all its environmental parameters and procedures for applying the information so gained to future projects of a similar nature. As things stand, the report's principal author noted, too many arguments about environmental impacts are based on prejudice rather than knowledge: "There are a lot of people on both side of the arguments who find it convenient not to know what actually happens when a project goes ahead. That way they can go into the next environmental battle with their positions unchanged."[47]

I have enumerated some of the more immediate public concerns and likely policy directions connected with the present global genetic transition, but those parts still do not quite add up to a whole. We need a way of looking at politics that sees public policy as a strategy for passing through a great period of change, of a sort that—even though it is largely of our creating—we do not fully comprehend or control. We also need to understand that the human species is going through a biological transition of its own, evident in new concerns about population and reproduction.

[5]

Human Lives,
Human Genes,
Human Numbers

TO MANY readers the foregoing matters may seem remote, the idea of a period of extensive global genetic change an abstract hypothesis of no immediate personal concern. And the proposition that we are present at the birth of a Biological Revolution may seem equally fanciful and distant from the daily reality of life. But there is another side to the evolutionary adventure, a parallel series of developments that is already transforming our own personal biological destinies, changing the rules that govern reproduction and birth, enabling us to make more choices—requiring us to do so, in fact—and raising new issues of social responsibility and personal freedom.

The Biological Revolution does more than create new kinds of power and responsibility in relation to plant and animal life; it also brings us inexorably closer to one of the most fearful of all evolutionary challenges—that of shaping the genetic evolution of the human species—and to confronting it as a political question. This is an issue that has arisen before, and the first time around it led to one of the most disastrous misuses of political power in all history.

The Birth of Eugenics

DR. ERASMUS DARWIN, the enthusiastic but premature promoter of evolution, had two grandsons who made a mark in the world. One, of course, was Charles Darwin. The other was Francis Galton, who founded the quasi-science known as eugenics.

Although Galton did not get around to coining the word "eugenics"—taken from a Greek root meaning "well born" or "noble in heredity"—until 1883, he laid out the theoretical foundations of his philosophy well before then. In fact, he had the idea in public circulation within the first decade after the publication of his cousin Charles' *Origin of Species*. The basic idea was both audacious and simple: He wanted to take evolution to its next logical step, from theory to practice, "to further the ends of evolution more rapidly and with less distress than if events were left to their own course." He proposed a deliberate program to improve the quality of the human stock.

Galton's ideas about how to breed genius were rather limited. As he presented them—first in a two-part magazine article, then in a book entitled *Hereditary Genius*—they were informed by a dubious method of research and saturated with a peculiarly English tendency to talk of human quality in the language of social class. His way of identifying people of natural ability was to consult reference books containing biographies of eminent men of the time, on the assumption that "high reputation is a pretty accurate test of high ability." As he studied the genealogies of

[149]

successful Englishmen he noted that they tended to be related to one another. He reasoned from this that families of reputation were more likely to produce offspring of ability. Staking a claim far to the heredity side of the heredity-environment spectrum, he concluded that "a man's natural abilities are derived by inheritance, under precisely the same limitations as are the form and physical features of the whole organic world."[1]

Armed with this insight, Galton began advocating a program to "produce a highly gifted race of men" who would be capable of leading the British Empire through the complexities of the coming twentieth century. He proposed government programs to discover the genetically superior young people and encourage them to marry one another. At first he recommended a non-coercive system of incentives and voluntary breeding, but after giving the matter more thought he decided it would be more effective for the state to rank people by ability and permit the highest-ranking people to have the most children. The middle orders could have medium-sized families and the lowest-ranked would be segregated in monasteries and convents, where they would be unable to reproduce at all.[2]

The strongest part of Galton's work was derived from his mathematical ability; he was a tireless collector of facts, and his accomplishments in figuring out patterns of mathematical relationship among aggregates of data are recognized as a major contribution to modern statistics.

The ideas of eugenics were taken up by people of oddly differing political orientations—conservative social Darwinists, radical free love proponents, Fabian Socialists such as George Bernard Shaw—but never had much effect on public policy in England. They did gain a small but secure foothold in the academic world. Galton, who was independently wealthy, endowed a Research Fellowship in National Eugenics at University College, London; after his death the bulk of his estate went to the College, which established a Department of Applied Statistics. This became the base of operations for Galton's most faithful disciple, Karl Pearson, and for Pearson's own intellectual creation, the science of biometrics.

Eugenics and biometrics remained a somewhat embattled minor school in the British scientific world. Pearson and his colleagues were often criticized for their extreme position on what had become widely known as the "nature-nurture" controversy; and biometrics was overshadowed by the rapid growth of genetics, the experimentally-based science derived from the work of Mendel. There was a bitter rivalry between the biometricians and the geneticists, and a corresponding personal feud between Pearson and the father of genetics, William Bateson. Bateson, who was such a strong admirer of Mendel's that he named his own son Gregory, thought the biometricians were seriously deficient in their grasp of the principles of heredity that Mendel had discovered.

The geneticists had several things working in their favor: One was a lack of interest in prescribing human breeding programs, which appeared to many to be crackpot politics. Another was the concept of recessive and dominant characteristics, which had much more analytical precision than prior vague notions about inheritance. Another was a laboratory approach which, using *Drosophila* and other fast-breeding species, soon amassed an impressive body of research tending to support and expand upon Mendel's hypotheses. And another was its concentration on the *genotype*, the genetic makeup of the organism, rather than the *phenotype*, the organism's observable characteristics; Bateson and his colleagues were moving directly toward a science of genetic information.

Galton's ideas did not really come into their own until they crossed the Atlantic; in the United States the eugenicists built a scientific empire beyond Galton's wildest dreams, and also opened up a whole new field of public policy.

Eugenicists in the New World were less troubled by the biometrics-genetics feud. William Davenport, Galton's most eminent American disciple, embraced Mendelian theory and incorporated it into his own work. He demonstrated a Mendelian basis for the inheritance of skin and eye color in humans, and built a school of eugenics that synthesized the two aproaches.

However, he shared with Galton and Pearson a strong tilt toward the nature side of the nature-nurture debate. He was certain that human intelligence and personal character were genetically inherited, and tended to describe all manner of things—including criminality, various mental deficiencies, and personal poverty—as though they were inherited in more or less the same way as eye color. He was strongly racist, after the manner of the times which equated race with national origin: He found Italians tending to crimes of personal violence; Jews prone to thievery; and Hungarians given to "larceny, kidnapping, assault, murder, rape, and sex-immorality."[3] He was also unconsciously sexist: He once wrote that love for the sea was a sex-linked recessive trait, since it showed up only in the male side of seagoing families.[4]

Davenport echoed Galton's advocacy of deliberate breeding to improve the human stock and sought to make genealogical information available to couples considering marriage so they could make sound biological decisions—

but he was far more deeply involved with the negative side of eugenics, the belief in the inheritability of disease, feeblemindedness, and criminality. His study of Mendelian genetics made him even more pessimistic than most eugenicists, since it led him to believe that undesirable characteristics would not be diluted by interbreeding with people of different stock but would persist in the society as recessive genes. "The idea of a 'melting-pot'," he wrote, "belongs to a pre-Mendelian age."[5]

These were explosive ideas in a country that had been settled by people of Anglo-Saxon stock and was now filling up with people from Eastern Europe and the Mediterranean regions. They had an impact far beyond the mild intellectual ripple that eugenics and biometry had caused in England.

Eugenic Politics

AMERICA'S gates swung open for eugenics. Lavish support came forth from the wealthy families and the great foundations. Davenport established a research center—the Station for the Experimental Study of Evolution—with a grant from the Carnegie Institution, and later added a Eugenics Record Office with grants from the Harriman and Rockefeller families. There was a Race Betterment Foundation at Battle Creek, Michigan, funded by cereal tycoon J. H. Kellogg, and—getting closer to the political agenda—a Committee to Study and Report on the Best Practical Means to Cut off the Supply of Defective Germ Plasm in the American Population.[6] Eugenics was taught in the universities; new findings were discussed at meetings of the American Eugenics Society and reported in the *Journal of Heredity*.

Eugenics was a mix of science and pseudo-science. As science, it had a growing body of data and statistical methodology, and produced solid findings on the inheritability of certain diseases; as pseudo-science it was a muddleheaded mess of racist and sexist prejudice, feeding into American paranoia about genetic contamination—a phenomenon that was in many ways quite similar to the witch hunts of the colonial era and the anti-Communist hysteria of the 1950s, and based on catastrophic scenarios much like those that surfaced during the biotechnology debates of the 1970s and 1980s. In this case the genetic threat was a flow of supposedly defective human germ plasm; the predicted outcome was a deterioration of American society marked by an increase in the populations of the prisons, the insane asylums, and the poorhouses. Although Davenport and his colleagues dutifully conceded that the new immigrant races contained much good stock, they were more outspoken on the subject of inferiority. The director of the Eugenics Record Offics testified to a congressional committed that: "The recent immigrants, as a whole, present a higher percentage of inborn socially inadequate qualities than do the older stocks."[7]

The eugenicists also worried about defective native stock. Intelligence tests were just coming into use in the United States and the man who first used them, Henry Goddard, wrote a widely read book entitled *The Kallikak Family: A Study in the Heredity of Feeble-mindedness*. The Kallikaks and the Jukes family (chronicled in other studies) vividly established the image of clans of shiftless, thieving, and overly fertile mental defectives.

In 1913, biologist H.E. Walker called on Americans to develop a "eugenic conscience" and outlined a political platform of legal measures to improve the quality of the nation's germ plasm: immigration restriction, tough marriage laws, and neuterization or sterilization "where necessary."[8] Actually, the incorporation of eugenic ideology into public policy was already well under way. Even before laws were passed to authorize it, male mental patients and criminals were being castrated and vasectomized, female inmates being sterilized by tubal ligation. In 1907 Indiana enacted the first sterilization law. Other states followed; by 1935 twenty states had authorized compulsory sterilization for certain crimes and many forms of mental illness, including alcoholism, and some 20,000 people had been legally sterilized.[9]

Under the same impetus, states passed laws restricting or voiding marriage among persons classed as "eugenically unfit." Some outlawed extramarital sexual relations among certain classes of unfit persons; some required a delay between the time of applying for a marriage license and the time of the wedding, a measure recommended by eugenecists as likely to discourage hasty unions of unfit persons. Most laws prohibiting or restricting interracial marriage also date from this period; 30 states passed miscegenation laws between 1915 and 1930.[10]

While the states passed sterilization and marriage laws, the federal government went to work on immigration, drawing heavily on the advice of eugenics experts. In 1917 Congress passed a law to exclude all illiterate Europeans over sixteen years of age. The impartial wording of the bill concealed its true intent, which was to reduce immigration from southern and eastern Europe, where literacy rates were low. (Earlier federal measures such as the Chinese Exclusion Act and the "Gentlemen's Agreement" with Japan had cut immigration from the Orient.) In 1921, amid increasing fear of a new postwar wave of immigrattion from Europe, Congress established the first quota system, limiting immigration from any nation to 3 percent of the number of persons of that nationality living in America in 1910. Three years later a more comprehensive law put a ceiling on immigration of approximately 150,000 per year. This was far fewer than the hundreds of thousands who had come over in the peak years; eugenics thus brought to an end the years of massive immigration, and imposed a temporary status quo on the racial makeup of American society.

The U.S. Supreme Court also did its part. State courts had declared several sterilization laws unconstitutional and eugenicists, looking for an opportunity to bring the issue before the Supreme Court, helped draw up a model law in Virginia and then found a good opportunity to test it. A young woman named Carrie Buck, daughter of an inmate of a state institution for the feeble-minded and herself classed as a moron according to IQ test performance, had given birth to a child before she was committed to the institution. The child—less than one year old—was examined by a eugenicist and pronounced below average; the institution's directors ordered that Carrie be sterilized under the law, which authorized it in cases where mental deficiency appeared in the third generation. A court-appointed guardian sued to block the operation, and the case went to the Supreme Court, which voted eight to one to uphold the Virginia statute. Justice Oliver Wendell Holmes declared, "Three generations of imbeciles are enough," and Carrie was sterilized. The child later died of an intestinal disorder, but her teachers believed her to be of above average intelligence.[11]

The eugenics movement peaked in the 1930s and then entered a period of decline. This has often been attributed to a reaction against the excesses of the Nazi regime in Germany, but it was more a gradual erosion of credibility, a loss of momentum during which eugenics faded temporarily from the prominent place it had occupied in the public dialogue.

For a while, it had been the very cutting edge of enlightened thought, enjoying the support of a long list of prominent Americans. It did have a recognizeable political identity—you were more likely to find the most enthusiastic eugenicists among racist conservatives and earnest believers in the infallibility of science—but people of many political persuasions believed it to contain a core of common sense and a hopeful vision of the future; there were liberal eugenicists and radical eugenicists. Even many of the opponents of eugenics shared a hope that human reproduction would in time be informed by more knowledge about genetics—but balked at the haste with which the reformers in America were enacting their dubious scientific conclusions into law. Bateson said: "It is not the tyrannical and capricious interference of a half-informed majority which can safely mould or purify a population."[12]

Gradually science accumulated a body of research indicating that matters were not as simple as the more strident eugenicists had portrayed them to be. Some of these findings came from people who were personally committed to the eugenics movement. One, Lionel Penrose, published a study showing that in the majority of cases mental deficiency was attributable to a multitude of causes of which genetic inheritance was only one element. He challenged the careless use of the word "feebleminded", and attacked the popular belief that there was a known genetic cause for mental illness. Other research dashed the fearful conviction that the numbers of defectives in the population were increasing, and undermined the eugenicists' plan to rid society of genetic undesirables through sterilization: It might be possible to reduce the incidence of diseases such as Huntington's chorea which were caused by dominant genes, but it would be a much trickier matter—probably quite impossible—to do anything about the numerous recessive genetic diseases.[13] Also, it had been made clear by the neo-Mendelians that, while there were indeed some physical characteristics attributable to a single gene, inheritance was a much more complex matter in which the interaction of many genes played a part: There was no hope of discovering the gene for altruism.

But even while eugenics was passing its prime in the United States and England, it was advancing to insane new heights in Germany. In the first year of Hitler's reign a eugenic sterilization program was proclaimed; it contained no hint of its future genocidal tendencies, but brought into being the first eugenic police state. It sought to root out a wide range of defects and disabilities that were believed to be hereditary—feeblemindedness, mental diseases, drug and alcohol addiction, bodily deformities. It set up a mandatory reporting procedure for doctors and a system of eugenic tribunals, and within three years had sterilized some 225,000 people.

Nazi eugenics did not immediately make common cause with anti-Semitism. For some years it was merely a heavy-handed program of genetic "improvement", with compulsory sterilzation of defectives and *Lebensborn* centers for delivering the healthy children of SS officers and other superior specimens. But by the late 1930s, when euthanasia of mental defectives was authorized, Jews were being automatically categorized as genetically inferior. It was an easy step from the executions of mental patients—soon being gassed in rooms disguised as showers—to the holocaust.

It took a long time before people outside of Germany realized what was happening there, and historians have had a hard time explaining why we were so resistant to discover the turn events had taken in a country that was not, after all, hermetically sealed from the outside world.[14] Although many reports came out of Germany and some were even printed in the newspapers, the human ability to resist information performed admirably; it was not until the war was over that the full story of the holocaust was accepted and comprehended. When it did become known, it revealed the madness and cruelty that the search for racial purity could produce, and established a connection between eugenics and genocide that still exists in the minds of many people.

Counselors and Screeners

EUGENICS ceased to reign as a political fad, a quick-fix approach to human progress. Many of its adherents distanced themselves from the cause, others worked to change its image, and the general public lost interest in it. Yet throughout the decades that the popularity of eugenics waned, the human race was not becoming any less responsible for evolution. On the contrary, the same growing body of scientific research that knocked the props out from under the first eugenics movement laid down the foundations for yet another one. The basic issues, far from having disappeared, are present among us still in even more complex forms.

Among the many research institutions endowed by true believers in the eugenic cause was the Dight Institute for

Human Genetics, established by a physician who left his estate to the University of Minnesota with the requirement that it be used "to promote biological race betterment." The will created a "heredity clinic," initially somewhat similar to other eugenics advice centers but with a growing emphasis on what its second director, Dr. Sheldon Reed, described as "a kind of genetic social work *without* eugenic connotations." [15] Genetic counseling, as Reed came to call his approach, included such simple matters as helping parents of defective children to overcome their feelings of personal guilt, and furnishing them with any information that might enable them to calculate the likelihood of another defective child and decide whether to have more children. In 1955 Reed published a textbook on genetic counseling which helped to establish the new field of practice.

For some years genetic counseling remained a minor specialty, of no great interest to the mainstream of American medicine—but gradually research established evidence of genetic factors in a number of diseases.

One of the first diseases to be clearly identified as genetic in origin was phenylketonuria (PKU), an inability to metabolize a certain amino acid, which leads to a toxic accumulation in the child's tissues and produces mental retardation. It became possible to identify this condition in babies and then to place them on a special diet, low in the critical amino, which would prevent the retardation.

Some states inaugurated programs to screen all newborn children for PKU, a policy that appeared to be not only humane and effective, but relatively inexpensive. At first this was done without any special legislative mandate, but then the cause of screening was taken up by state chapters of the National Association for Retarded Children, and during the 1960s it advanced rapidly: In 1965, the peak year, 29 states passed laws to create PKU screening programs.[16]

The early eugenicists had been wrong in their belief that various forms of criminality were caused by a single gene, but PKU appears to be one of a large class of disorders that actually *are* traceable to a dominant gene, a sex-linked gene, or two recessive genes. By 1971 geneticists had identified some 900 such disorders and about a thousand more were believed to be in the same category.[17] Some of these could be identified by postnatal testing programs similar to those used for PKU and some could be treated if identified.

While the scope of postnatal testing expanded, other forms of genetic detective work were also being developed. One was prenatal amniocentesis—analysis of fluid drawn from the amniotic sac in the uterus of a pregnant woman. The other was testing of prospective parents to find if they were carriers of genetic disorders.

And while the techniques improved, the whole matter became more politically explosive. In 1967 an act of the British Parliament granted the right to legal abortion for, among other causes, likelihood that the child would be born with a serious handicap. In 1973, in the case of *Roe v. Wade*, the U.S. Supreme Court established the right to abortion. Coming at the same time as advances in amniocentesis, these developments enabled parents to abort a fetus if it was found to have one of the detectable genetic disorders or a chromosomal disorder such as Down's syndrome. The number of legal abortions rose rapidly, and the anti-abortion movement arose in opposition.

Another political development emerged with the news that some of the detectable disorders had strong connections to certain ethnic groups. There was some evidence that this was because the disorders had survival value in the regions in which they originated.[18] Sickle-cell anemia, for example, appears to be not only a disease but also a form of biochemical resistance against malarial parasites common in Africa. Other genetic disorders with similar ethnic allegiances were Tay-Sachs disease, higher among Ashkenazic Jews; and Cooley's anemia (thalassemia), found among people of Mediterranean origin.

As these connections became known to the public and its representatives, ethnic groups began advocating screening programs for their specific disorders. Black leaders sponsored sickle-cell screening laws in several states and backed the National Sickle Cell Anemia Control Act, which was passed by Congress in 1972.

Italians took an interest in Cooley's anemia, and attempted to tack it onto the sickle-cell bill. When that failed, Representative Robert Giaimo of Connecticut and several other Congressmen introduced a bill that became the National Cooley's Anemia Control Act. Senator Jacob Javits of New York responded with a National Tay-Sachs Control Act but was eventually persuaded that legislating genetic screening policy one disease at a time was not the best way to go about it. Tay-Sachs was instead incorporated into the National Genetic Diseases Act, passed in 1976.

By that time it was becoming apparent that screening programs presented problems as well as benefits to the affected minority groups.

The first state sickle-cell laws were especially weak: They failed to distinguish between sickle-cell trait, which is related to sickle-cell anemia but is not a disease, and the more serious disorder. In some cases they confused sickle-cell anemia with diseases capable of being prevented by immunization or treated by diet, like PKU. Some classified it as a communicable disease.

Also, there were unanticipated social consequences. Sometimes sickle-cell testing raised questions about a child's paternity and caused serious family conflicts. The new problem of "genetic discrimination" arose when insurance companies began raising premiums on sickle-cell carriers, the armed forces considered rejecting them, and some airlines grounded black employees because of the effects of high altitude on persons with sickle-cell trait.

The federal laws were in part extensions of genetic screening and in part reforms of some of the more serious abuses of it. The National Sickle Cell Control Act of 1972 and the Genetic Diseases Act of 1976 both mandated high scientific standards for screening programs, required that they be voluntary, and prevented them from being linked to eligibility for other federal sources.

By the late 1970s genetic screening had become a recognized part of medical practice and public policy and an accepted part of modern life for many people. A considerable amount of social learning had taken place, both in regard to genetic disorders and what could be done about them, and also in regard to the new problem of genetic discrimination. It had become generally accepted that genetic screening should be accompanied by genetic counseling—which is ideally a humanized feedback system to give people information about the situations they are dealing with and the choices that are available. If screening and counseling belong to the Biological Revolution, they also have dual citizenship in the Information Revolution. Indeed, one of the many political questions is that of storage of genetic data—who should have access to it, how its confidentiality should be protected. In yet another way, genetic information becomes symbolic information.

Moving alongside the growing body of information about genetic disorders—indeed, inseparable from it—is a growing body of information about other factors that influence the health and survival prospects of newborn infants. Knowledge about the effects of nutrition, about smoking and alcohol consumption by pregnant women, about environmental conditions and chemicals that can affect the genes of an adult before conception or the health of a fetus; all this comprises part of the reality of parenthood in the modern world, part of humanity's unavoidable responsibility for its own evolution.

The Politics of the Gene Screen

ALTHOUGH genetic screening and counseling have evolved rapidly, both are in their infancy. In the near future, science will be able to perform the "total gene screen"— that is, to analyze a person's entire genome and produce a complete genetic profile, identifying all abnormal genes and chromosomes. This will probably be an automated process, a joint product of biological science and information technology: A programmed machine will process blood samples and print out the results.[19]

Another quantum leap, another Pandora's box of hopes and headaches. It means that a person will be able to know if, for example, he or she possesses a gene that carries a high likelihood of heart disease in middle age. That is not exactly good news, but it enables the person to begin early to take steps—such as going on a low-fat diet—that will lessen the chance of an early death from an unexpected heart attack. In many ways, such testing may reveal problems that can be treated or cured.

But genetic screening may reveal a disease for which there is no treatment or cure. It is already possible, for example, to identify a DNA marker that indicates a high likelihood the person carries what is sometimes called "Woody Guthrie's disease"—which promises a future of madness, suffering and painful death.[19]

Genetic screening can identify hypersusceptibility—genetically inherited vulnerability to certain chemicals, such as asbestos, in the environment. This is a central part of a new science, ecogenetics, dealing with the relationship between an organism's genetic makeup and its environment. It can predict who is likely to be harmed—to develop cancer, anemia, dermatitis or other ailment—from being in the presence of a certain substance such as asbestos or pesticides. It offers a far more precise understanding of such problems than is to be found in the present debate over "safe levels" of such substances, because it is clear that what may be safe for one person can be fatally dangerous to another.

This is a tremendous advance in knowledge; one science writer said it "could be the greatest advance in disease protection since Edward Jenner's work on vaccination in the late 18th century."[20] But genetic screening to obtain such information is opposed by various groups who, depending on their political orientation, view it as sexist, racist, anti-labor, elitist, paternalistic, or an invasion of privacy. All the problems that arose around sickle-cell anemia arise again, this time along a much broader front.

The opposition from women's groups has to do with the higher vulnerability of a fetus to some chemicals in the workplace, which has resulted in women being refused certain jobs. The opposition from organized labor stems from the fear that employers will screen out hypersusceptibles and relax efforts to clean up workplace pollutants. Some people of a more conservative bent prefer to stay with the basic idea that some jobs are risky, you take your chances and get good pay; others contend that such risks always involve costs that sooner or later are paid by society. Many people just don't like the idea of so much intimate *knowledge* being available, and fear that it will be misused—by industries, by government, by the individuals themselves. Again we confront the need to know, and the fear of knowing.

The advance in gene screening will produce much controversy, much resistance from people who really don't want to deal with such knowledge, probably some abuses and also better lives for many people. It will change the ways many things are done, and it will change us, as we deal with a new body of knowledge.

And while it does, other lines of development along the human genetic front progress also. One of the major ones is in human reproductivity: It expands the options for couples who wish to have a child but, because (as a result of whatever knowledge they have about their own genetic heritage) they believe that there is a high likelihood of its inheriting a genetic disorder, choose to conceive it some other way—through artificial insemination or one of the other methods of conception that science is inventing as it goes about the business of changing the rules of human conception and birth.

Babies in the Brave New World

WHEN THE eugenics movement was on the rise in England, Aldous Huxley observed it from his vantage point as a member of an eminent scientific family, and satirized it in *Brave New World*. The opening scene in Huxley's novel was a visit to the Central London Hatchery, where human eggs were fertilized in test tubes and the embryos cultivated in large bottles until they were ready to be "decanted" into life. It was imagery of mythic proportions, and a setback to eugenics no less serious than the new discoveries of the geneticists and the genocidal madness of the Hitler years; it vividly linked the eugenic cause with an unfeeling subordination of individual human life to social purposes.

Brave New World was satire, not prophecy. We are not gestating babies in bottles, and I doubt that we ever will. But we are well into a new era in human reproduction, a startling transformation in which the most profound and personal aspects of our biological functioning are carried out with the assistance of scientists, entrepreneurs of the Biological Revolution, and anonymous human beings.

Artificial insemination, now commonplace among animal breeders, is rapidly becoming an equally familiar part of the reproductive repertoire of human beings. Artificial insemination by donor is routinely resorted to in situations where the husband is infertile, or where genetic screening indicates the likelihood that a child will be born with a congenital disorder resulting from recessive genes in both parents or from a dominant gene in the father. Artificial insemination by donor can be psychologically difficult for the husband, but the stress seems to be lessening as the procedure becomes more commonplace. A doctor in a New York fertility research institution was recently quoted as saying: "A lot of things we wouldn't do a few years ago, we no longer think twice about. For instance, I do 40 or 50 artificial inseminations a week, whereas a few years ago we would do 10 or 12 a year. The repellant connotations of artificial insemination are almost non-existent now. Couples not only accept it but seem to regard it as more natural than adoption."[21]

Human artificial insemination has arrived among us quietly—has been on its way for a good two centuries since the first successful artificial inseminations of animals were performed. The other major entry into the new world of human reproductivity came more suddenly: The news flashed from England in 1978 that the first "test tube baby" had been born. Actually, Louise Brown did not begin her existence in a test tube, but in a flat petri dish, resembling an ashtray, which is commonly used for *in vitro* fertilization. The eggs are removed from the mother and fertilized in the dish with the husband's sperm. The embryo grows for a few days in a nutrient solution, inside an incubator which keeps it at the temperature of a human body, then it is implanted in the mother's uterus—an instrument of far more technological sophistication than Huxley's glass bottles. The embryo develops naturally in the mother's womb and makes a thoroughly traditional transition to the world at the appropriate time, and differs from other babies only in having been out there before.

The development of a workable method of *in vitro* fertilization made it possible for women who had been unable to conceive to bear children. As other related techniques are developed, a whole range of mix-and-match variations on parenthood present themselves: If the father is infertile, the egg can be fertilized by sperm from a donor. If the mother is unable to carry a child, the embryo can be implanted in a surrogate mother. The much simpler technique of artificially inseminating a surrogate mother (in cases where the husband is fertile but the wife unable to conceive or carry a child) has already made its debut.

Time ran a cover story on "The New Science of Conception" not long ago; it included a sidebar about a pretty young New Jersey housewife who agreed, for a fee of $10,000, to serve as a surrogate mother for a couple who were unable to conceive a child and had been discouraged by the delays and expenses involved in adopting one. The article mentioned that some surrogate parenting agencies insist that there be no personal contact between the parents and the biological mother of their child, while in other instances a close friendship develops; in one case, the couple named their new daughter after the surrogate mother and she occasionally visited the child toward whom she felt like "a loving aunt".[22] Surrogate motherhood carries its own load of social/political issues—there is the matter of drawing up a tight contract, since sometimes the mother refuses to give up the child, and a fair number of people regard the whole thing as immoral—but I suspect it is here to stay.

Embryo transplant, also first perfected in animal breeding, offers yet another variation: If the mother is able to carry a child but unable to conceive it, another woman is artificially inseminated and, five days after fertilization, the embryo is removed and implanted in the mother, where it then develops as though it were her own. The first child was born by this method in January 1984. Another technique removes eggs surgically from an "egg donor", fertilizes one (or more) *in vitro*, then implants it in the mother.

Like other methods of artificial conception, embryo transplant serves people who carry genetic disorders as well as those with infertility or physical disability. About 40 percent of the women who applied for embryo transplants when the process was first becoming available did so because they were concerned about passing on genetically transferred disease.[23] Eventually the embryo transfer process may replace amniocentesis; the embryo will be removed from the womb, tested, and then reimplanted in the same mother.

It is possible to freeze semen or human embryos, and this development has given rise to some strange new biopolitical developments. In France a man died after having deposited sperm in a sperm bank, and his widow asked for it in order to be impregnated and give the man a posthumous offspring. The bank refused, saying the sperm was the dead man's property and he had left no instructions on what to do with it. The widow sued the sperm bank and, after some bizarre courtroom debate over whether the sperm was part of the man's estate or part of his own body, it was awarded to his wife who announced that she planned to conceive a child with it. (She tried, but did not succeed.) In a more publicized case, a couple died, leaving behind, in Australia, two artificially fertilized embryos. There was some talk of destroying the embryos, but right-to-life groups intervened and sought to have a legal guardian appointed for them. A right-to-life attorney from Los Angeles thought they might be heirs to the husband's sizeable estate until it was learned that they had been conceived with ova from the deceased woman and sperm from an anonymous donor. The Australians settled the matter with a new law providing that embryos could be "adopted" and implanted in some mother-to-be.

Perhaps the strongest indicator that we have indeed entered a new world is the sudden obsolescence of the vocabulary concerning parenthood. Alexander Capron, a law professor who specializes in legal matters concerning the new biotechnologies, remarked to a Congressional science subcommittee that "Many of the new reproductive possibilities remain so novel that terms are lacking to describe the human relationships they can create."[24] Certainly it is inadequate to describe the situation of an embryo adopted and then born to a woman to whom it has no genetic relationship, both its own parents deceased before it had even entered the womb of the person who will be its legal mother. Our most familiar and emotion-tinged designations—such as "mother" and "father"—need to be qualified by modifications such as "biological" and "legal", and even those are not always up to defining the precise nature of the relationship.

Some people see the biotechnologies as new weaponry in the battle of the sexes. I recently came across a book by a feminist writer who charges that "the technology is male-dominated and buttresses male power over women"— that it produces not new choices for women but only new avenues for "control by men of female biological reproductive processes."[25] At the same time, some male observers fear that the new methods render the human father obsolete by enabling women to have children without any direct contact with males. There is a feminist sperm bank in California; the majority of its clients are single women, and over a third are lesbians. Coming into a society in which feminism is a potent political force, the family an institution with its back to the wall, and all social roles in flux, the new reproductive technologies offer further reason not to expect a stable future.

Taking Care of Baby Doe

THERE IS yet another area of human reproductivity that has recently become a matter of public concern and government policy. This is the one that broke into the mass media in the spring of 1982 with the case of "Baby Doe."

Neither Baby Doe's name nor that of his parents has ever been made public, but the basic facts of the incident have been extensively documented. A woman in Bloomington, Indiana, mother of two healthy children, gave birth to a defective male child. He was a Down's syndrome baby and also had serious deformities of the esophagus: an atresia (in which the esophagus comes to a dead end so that no food can reach the stomach through it), and a fistula (the lower end of the interrupted esophagus hooked directly into the windpipe so that breathing is difficult and the lungs are eventually "digested" by the stomach juices).[26]

Baby Doe's parents were presented with clear choices about what to do. Some physicians recommended what they called a "full-court press": immediate transfer of the baby to an Indianapolis hospital, surgery to repair the esophagus, and a battery of tests to determine what other malformations it might have. (The baby had been blue at birth, and might have an enlarged heart.) The doctor who had delivered the baby suggested an alternative: They could refuse to consent to the surgery. In the latter case, the baby would die of pneumonia in a few days. The parents chose the latter course, and were soon in the center of a huge controversy of modern biopolitics.

The child was kept in the hospital under a clearly specified treatment program. He could be fed orally, but hospital personnel were advised that such feeding might result in aspiration and death; intravenous feeding was forbidden; and he should be kept comfortable and given sedation as needed.

Meanhile, a series of legal developments unfolded. First, a hearing before a superior court judge, who ruled that, since there were two divergent medical opinions, the parents could select whichever one they chose; this meant that the child would be permitted to die.

Right-to-life activists soon learned of the decision. There followed another hearing, a series of legal maneuvers, a sudden flood of national publicity. Appeals to the White House and the Supreme Court were in the works when, in the sixth day of his life, Baby Doe died. The child's death did not, however, end the controversy that had grown up around the case. A few days later attention focused on a child born with a severe form of spina bifida, its spinal cord protruding through an opening in the lower back. There had been reports that the parents refused to authorize surgery, but then other arrangements were made: The child would receive surgery and be adopted. President Reagan sent a memo to the Secretary of Health and Human Services instructing him to enunciate a strong federal policy in regard to such cases, and the Department responded by sending out a warning to all health care providers that they faced the loss of federal funds if they denied treatment or nourishment to any handicapped baby.

Early the following year, the Reagan administration made public a set of directives that became known as the "Baby Doe regulations." They required hospitals to post notices warning employees of their obligation to feed and care for handicapped infants, and set up a hotline to make it possible for people to inform the federal government of violations. In response to such confidential calls, "Baby Doe squads" of federal officials began to investigate hospitals, and a new chapter of American political history began. An administration dedicated to ending "big brother" government had established a conspicuous presence in the delivery wards and thereby taken on a new role as "big mother," guarantor of every infant's right to the fullest capabilities of modern medicine.

Since then, amid much pulling and tugging between different political factions and branches of government, that policy has been somewhat modified. The American Medical Association and the American Hospital Association brought a suit against the Department of Health and Human Services and won it when a federal court struck down the Baby Doe regulations as a violation of parents' right to privacy and of doctors' duty of confidentiality to patients. Another Baby Doe case made the headlines when a couple in New York refused surgical closure of a spinal defect in their baby girl who had been born with a number of defects including spina bifada and hydrocephaly. Right-to-life groups soon became involved, as did the Department of Justice. The courts rejected various attempts to compel the parents to order the spinal operation. The parents did agree to various treatment procedures including a shunt operation to drain fluid from the baby's head. When the baby was six months old, they took her home.[27] That same year (1984) Congress passed, and President Reagan signed, a bill making it unlawful to withold "medically indicated treatment" but excepting cases where surgery would be unlikely to save the child or be futile or inhumane. The White House continued to be strongly interested in such cases and right-to-life groups continued to be vigilantly on guard against denials of surgery by parents of defective children, but a full-court press was no longer federally mandated in all cases.

The issue has arisen for the same set of reasons that other biopolitical issues have arisen: Technology has changed the rules. In this case, it is medical technology—advances in drug therapy, intensive care, transfusion techniques, surgery, anesthesia and radiotherapy; and a great increase in knowledge about birth defects and treatment. As a result, it is now possible to save babies that would certainly have died a few decades ago. Some of these babies grow up to lead more or less satisfying and productive lives, and some of them remain severely handicapped, condemned to years of pain, paralysis, incontinence, mental retardation and repeated surgery.

Choices have to be made: choices to use all the technology, or choices to withold it or use it selectively. An English physician reports on a long period of time during which his hospital followed a policy of "non-selective treatment." All available methods were used in all cases, for a thirteen year period from 1958 to 1971; his conclusion and that of the hospital administration was that, "in spite of a progressively increasing survival rate the problems we created were greater than we solved. Treating all babies without selection resulted in massive suffering for the largest number in spite of massive cost to the community." They adopted a policy of selective treatment to give treatment to children who "had a chance of a life with a moderate handicap" (defined to include such conditions as absence of bladder or rectal sphincter control, partial paralysis, partial absence of skin sensation, or moderate hydrocephalus), and to deny treatment to children judged "certain to suffer from severe handicaps." Denial of treatment meant a decision to permit the baby to die.[28]

Those are hard decisions to make, and they are made by fallible human beings. They can be wrong; children who would have had decent lives might be permitted to die, children might be saved at great effort for lifetimes of suffering, immense financial cost of repeated surgery and high-technology care, and enormous stress for parents and siblings. They are also, as are all matters that influence survival and reproduction, evolutionary decisions—especially so in that parents of defective babies often choose not to have any more children. But once the technology exists, the choices have to be made—either to use it or not to use it. These are moral choices, and for many reasons—including the public cost of care for handicapped persons and the question of the rights of the child and the parents—political decisions as well.

Comparable technological progress is being made in the care of premature babies, and raising the same kinds of issues. Only a few years ago, doctors might try hard to save the life of a child weighing three pounds, but one weighing two pounds would be allowed to die on the assumption that it could not be saved by any effort. Today babies born three to three and a half months premature, some weighing little more than one pound, are routinely saved and further progress in the same direction can be expected. One way to look at this is to note that it is yet another reduction in the time it is necessary for a child to be in the womb—since it can be conceived in the laboratory and end what would be its natural gestation period in a neonatal intensive care unit—and can thus be seen as movement toward ectogenesis: growing the human fetus in an artificial womb. I have my doubts about this development, but some people take it very seriously and understand its political implications. The feminist writer Shulamith Firestone strongly advocated it as "the freeing of women from the tyranny of their reproductive biology," displacing the childbearing effort to society as a whole,[29] and the Australian ethicists Peter Singer and Deane Wells suggest it as one way of ending the abortion problem, since embryos could be removed from the wombs of women who did not want them, kept alive and, as children, eventually be given up for adoption.[30]

The Legal Wilderness

AS A FAITHFUL reader of "Dear Abby," I am struck by the frequency of letters about the etiquette and ethics of adoption. Most of the drama that finds its way into the paper concerns the adoptive child's curiosity about his or her biological parents. The child, usually sometime in the early adult years, goes off in search of his or her "real" mother or father. Often this causes great stress to the adoptive parents; sometimes it causes other kinds of family upheaval, as in the cases where the biological parent would just as soon not take on the emotional ordeal of greeting an adult who was given up for adoption as a baby.

There are many variations on the theme, and as I read such letters I muse about the "Dear Abby" of twenty years hence, when the children of *in vitro* fertilization, artificial insemination, embryo freezing, and surrogate motherhood grow up and start asking questions. It should make interesting reading.

Undoubtedly there will be complications, and probably some serious personal problems—but the human animal is an adaptable creature and I doubt that the emotional tangles of the future will be any more perplexing than the legal tangles of the present, as the first parents of the Biological Revolution try to make their way through a legal system that is equipped to deal with (a) normal parenthood, and (b) adoption—and not much else.

[177]

There are about a quarter of a million children alive in the United States today who were conceived by artificial insemination by donor. Their legal status in society and that of their parents is now becoming fairly clearly defined, but it was tough going in the early years. In 1921, the first time the matter came up before the courts, a husband in a Canadian divorce case argued that his wife, who had conceived a child through artificial insemination by donor, was guilty of adultery. The Canadian court did not give a definite ruling on that issue, but an Illinois court did in 1954. The court said: "Artificial insemination (by donor), with or without the consent of the husband, is contrary to public policy and good morals, and constitutes adultery on the part of the mother. A child so conceived is not a child born in wedlock and is therefore illegitimate."[31] Since then many cases have come before the courts, raising questions about the legitimacy of the child, the morality of the mother, and the rights and obligations of the father— such as whether he is required to support the child after a divorce, and whether he has visitation rights. Gradually the legal system is moving toward recognition that, when husband and wife have agreed to conceive a child through artificial insemination by donor, the child is legitimate, the husband is its legal father, and the mother is not entitled to a scarlet letter—but the progress is gradual indeed, and many more disputes will be aired in court and more bills drafted in the state capitols before government catches up with this relatively simple facet of the Biological Revolution.

There are far fewer *in vitro*-conceived children among us at present, but their number is growing despite the extremely precarious legality of the *in vitro* process. Many states have laws, passed after the U.S. Supreme Court's

1973 *Roe v. Wade* decision allowing abortion, that prohibit or limit experimentation with fetuses. These could quite possibly be used to prosecute anyone performing an *in vitro* fertilization if the court were persuaded that the process itself—or the freezing of embryos which is sometimes an adjunct to it—constituted experimentation.

Surplus embryos present another delicate issue: When an *in vitro* fertilization is to be attempted, the doctor commonly gives the mother a drug to induce "super-ovulation," and a number of eggs are removed from her ovaries at the same time; these are fertilized en masse and there are likely to be many embryos left over: little specks of tissue that have the unsettling potential of becoming human beings. Sometimes these are frozen for a later implantation attempt if the first one does not take (this was how the orphaned embryos in Australia had come to be), and sometimes they are simply destroyed. Sometimes they are used in scientific research, which again raises the spectre of experimentation with human life. It is possible that in the near future they will be preserved and offered for "adoption". The director of the Mayo Clinic's fertility department in Rochester, Minnesota told the newspapers that this approach "has a lot more going for it than adopting babies after birth."[32]

Of all the items in the new reproductive toolkit, surrogate motherhood seems to be the most difficult for people to accept. A commission created by the British Parliament in 1982 to propose policies for the new reproductive technologies was quite willing to permit research with embryos up to 14 days old, but recommended outlawing surrogate motherhood because it would be "liable to moral objection."[33] The legal status of the surrogate mother is, to say the least, insecure: Some states make it a crime to accept payment for giving up a child for adoption, which is what a surrogate mother more or less does. Most states have no laws that apply to surrogate motherhood and the whole transaction is subject to contractual agreement between the surrogate mother and the prospective parents—except that there is some doubt as to whether such contracts will be honored by the courts. As of this writing some states are considering laws to permit and regulate surrogate motherhood, others are considering laws to outlaw it completely; this suggests that in the future couples who want to become parents through that particular method and who can afford to do so will do what people of means always do in such situations—travel to the place where the legal situation is favorable to whatever they want to do.

A philosophy professor, testifying before a Congressional subcommittee, called the present array of legal arrangements "a patchwork of laws and gaps, stigmas, deprivations, uncertainties, confusions and fears."[34] The legislators are hard at work creating what amounts to a whole new legal system for a new era in human parenthood: They will have to determine the legal status of embryos and of children born from the various new technologies, referee the rights and obligations of various combinations of biological and legal parents, decide what to do about the non-conventionals—single people, homosexual couples, transsexuals, and others—who claim a right to become parents, and do the whole thing in a context of continuing change as present methods are improved and new ones developed. The issue of patenting will arise again and again in relation to these methods, and so will the larger evolutionary question that has never been disposed of—

responsibility for the genetic future of the human species itself.

Eugenics II

ALDOUS HUXLEY, who satirized eugenics in *Brave New World*, understood that the eugenicists with their cheerfully authoritarian programs for improving the species were not the only ones influencing the course of human evolution. In *Brave New World Revisited* he wrote about the other side of the coin: dysgenics, the deterioration of the gene pool brought about as an accidental by-product of human progress.

In this second half of the twentieth century we do nothing systematic about our breeding; but in our random and unregulated way we are not only over-populating our planet, we are also, it would seem, making sure that these greater numbers shall be of biologically poorer quality. In the bad old days children with considerable, or even with slight, hereditary defects rarely survived. Today, thanks to sanitation, modern pharmacology and the social conscience, most of the children born with hereditary defects reach maturity and multiply their kind. Under the conditions now prevailing, every advance in medicine will tend to be offset by a corresponding advance in the survival rate of individuals cursed by some genetic insufficiency. In spite of new wonder drugs and better treatment (indeed, in a certain sense, precisely because of these things), the physical health of the general population will show no improvement, and may even deteriorate.[35]

Genetic screening and genetic counseling are the respectable modern descendants of the eugenics movement—but in practice their impact may be either eugenic or dysgenic, may lessen or increase the sum total of genetic defect in the human gene pool. If a woman has an amniocentesis and discovers she is carrying a fetus with a genetic defect and aborts it, she and her husband may then conceive again and safely produce a number of children who do not have the defect—but who carry the recessive genes for it. This would have only a minute short-term impact on the gene pool, but after fifty generations it could increase the number of carriers of the recessive gene for cystic fibrosis, for example, by fifty percent.[36]

The same couple might choose to conceive by means of artificial insemination or an egg donor. This is what some writers have hailed as the "new eugenics," based on information and personal choice rather than social coercion.[37] As more information and reproductive alternatives become available, the cumulative effect will probably have a far greater eugenic payoff than did the first round of eugenic policies and practices—i.e., vasectomizing alcoholics and putting immigration quotas on Hungarians.

And there are other eugenic forces at work. In Japan there has been a rapid reduction in the number of children per family, accelerated by a 1948 "eugenic protection law" which legalized abortion and provided further public support to family planning. Japanese scientists predict several eugenic side-effects including a reduction in the percentage of children born with chromosomal defects (such as Down's) that are associated with older mothers, and fewer of the serious Rh diseases which increase with the number of children the mother has born.[38] An American study group, the Committee on Population Growth and the

American Future, came to similar conclusions about the eugenic effect of family planning.

One should not assume, however, that eugenics in the future will be entirely a matter of voluntary decisions made by parents or felicitous by-products of family planning. On the contrary, there is every reason to expect that government agencies will launch deliberate eugenics programs. Again, Japan may be a harbinger: Public health authorities there lauched a program aimed at Duchenne muscular dystrophy: screening, amniocentesis, and abortion. They expect it to reduce the incidence of that disease by more than 12 percent in one generation.[39] This is technically a voluntary program, since the decision to abort is the mother's, but an element of coercion is undoubtedly present; one cannot imagine too many Japanese women choosing to buck the social current.

Whenever couples turn to such methods for genetic reasons—because they do not want to produce a defective child or because they do not want to contribute defective genes to future generations—they naturally expect that the donated sperm or egg will be at least free of genetic defects, and preferably from a healthy and intelligent person. Like any prospective parents they hope to have a healthy child and would not mind bringing a superior human being into the world.

The beginnings of artificial insemination by donor were, like the beginnings of many things, haphazard. Most of the donors were medical students and usually some effort was made to match them up—in terms of general physical characteristics—with the legal father. No doubt the doctors who oversaw such programs regarded it as inherently eugenic, but over the long haul it is doubtful that a program of breeding a race of medical students would bear up under close public scrutiny.

As the technology of genetic screening advances, it becomes commonplace to test sperm and egg donors carefully. This decreases (but does not eliminate) the possibility that a genetic defect may be carried in donated material. It also provides the rationale for governmental involvement; wherever states and national governments recognize the legality of the new reproductive methods, they generally establish licensing procedures and regulations, and eugenic considerations—or dysgenic ones—again become issues of public policy.

Public officials are reluctant to confront the evolutionary issues raised by the new reproductive technologies—the uncomfortable but inevitable fact that any decision which determines the source of donated genetic material will have impacts for generations to come. But the connection is obvious and is being expressed forthrightly in the private sector.

The best-known enterprise in this field is the offspring—although of questionable legitimacy—of Hermann Muller, one of the pioneering figures in genetics. Muller, an American, was a member of the group that made the exhaustive studies of the fast-breeding *Drosophila* fly that laid down the basis of neo-Mendelian genetics. He went on to experiments using x-rays to induce mutations in flies (a body of work that one scientist called "a decisive advance in man's probing of nature—the first time that he had willfully changed the hereditary material"), which eventually won him a Nobel prize.[40] He worked for a time in the Soviet Union under the great plant geneticist N.I. Vavilov, the man who had classified the world's centers of natural genetic diversity.

Muller was opposed to the eugenics movement in its original form—in the late 1940s, when its time seemed to have passed, he warned that it represented "a continuing peril, to be vigilantly guarded against"—but he was also worried about the dysgenic effects of modern science. He saw likely deterioration of the human gene pool not only from social and medical advances, but also from the effects of increased radiation—a subject he understood as well as anyone alive. He warned that what he called the "genetic load"—the total amount of defective material in the human gene pool—might well increase to the point where future generations would be able to do little more than doctor themselves.[41]

Muller, like many other genetic scientists, found that his concerns about the deterioration of the gene pool led him finally toward thoughts of deliberate improvement. In 1954 he said: "The fact that the so-called eugenics of the past was so mistaken . . . is no more argument against eugenics as a general proposition than, say, the failure of democracy in ancient Greece is a valid argument against democracy in general."[42] His own concept of a new approach was what he called "germinal choice." He thought couples should have access to banks containing the sperm of men of superior physical health and/or intellect, so that they could have the opportunity, to, as he put it, "bestow on themselves children with a maximal chance of being highly endowed, and also to make them an exemplary contribution to humanity."[43]

Muller set out to establish a sperm bank based on the "germinal choice" idea, and obtained the support of Robert K. Graham, a wealthy inventor-businessman from Southern California. It was an unlikely alliance—biopolitics makes strange bedfellows—between Muller, an old-school idealistic Socialist, and the right-wing millionaire: Muller saw germinal choice as a way toward a classless society of healthy and altruistic human beings, and Graham saw it as a way to beef up America's population of scientific geniuses. Muller broke off with Graham, but after he died Graham went ahead and founded the Repository for Germinal Choice, announcing that its stock in trade would be sperm donated by Nobel prizewinners. Among the donors was William Shockley—inventor of the transistor, proponent of vintage 1920 eugenics views on racial inferiority, and advocate of sterilization for people of low IQ. Graham predicted to a *Time* reporter that the children of the Repository would "sail through schools."[44]

I personally find the prospect of a race of Shockleys no more inspiring than that of a race of medical students, but the essence of the new eugenics of germinal choice is that people are free to do things which seem to them to be contributions to the future of the human species— and may not seem so to others. Human reproduction does not become the totally state-directed hatching operation envisioned in *Brave New World*, but remains a matter of personal choice leavened with the ever-present reality of social pressure. This does not mean that there has been no change. On the contrary, the basic dimensions of biological procreation are changing as parents begin to draw on a wider selection of genetic information in the conception of children. The circle of family widens through space and time. There has always been adoption, and in recent years this has become another global information exchange, with agencies finding children in distant countries. The new technologies enable sperm and embryos to travel about the world—and, frozen, to travel through time also.

Hermann Muller called this "eutelegenesis:" long-distance eugenics.

The new technologies also increase the likelihood of large numbers of offspring from a single parent. Through sperm banking and artificial insemination a man can have as many offspring as a prize bull, and *in vitro* fertilization creates the possibility of large numbers of children from one mother.

These are not imaginings about the far distant future. Graham's sperm bank has been doing business in Southern California for some years now; when he was interviewed by *Time* in 1984 it had already brought fifteen children into the world. And more are on the way.

The Uncertainties of Freedom

EVOLUTION is learning, but learning is not mere accumulation of information. We also have to learn what can be done with information, and what it does to us. Some of this comes hard. There is no tougher evolutionary lesson than the discovery that scientific information is always partial, and that human progress is not what we had secretly hoped it would be—namely, the gaining of a great range of choice together with relief from the fear that some of our choices might turn out to be the wrong ones. We learn instead that more knowledge only takes us into new landscapes of uncertainty.

Every day, people make decisions that bring children into the world—or do not—and contribute to the genetic future of the species. Those decisions are based on ideas about what constitutes a superior or a defective human being, but the ideas are notoriously difficult to dignify as facts.

[187]

It all seemed so easy to Francis Galton as he browsed through *Men of the Time*. He had no doubt that the illustrious gentlemen who graced its pages represented the cream of the human gene pool, and he was equally certain such "natural ability" was something that, as he put it, "a modern European possesses in a much greater average share than men of the lower races."[45] He held it to be self-evident that the best specimens of *Homo sapiens* were successful English males of the educated classes—i.e., people rather like himself—and he thus fell prey to the occupational disease of eugenicists: unconscious ethnocentrism.

Galton's followers, eugenicists of the twentieth century, looked for some source of data more scientifically presentable than the directories of famous men, and found it in intelligence testing. It is not surprising that the histories of eugenics and IQ measurement are closely intertwined. Eugenics had to have something—preferably something quantifiable—which could serve as an index of human superiority.

When Alfred Binet, the father of IQ testing, began his research into this subject he did so with the conviction that the best measurement of intelligence was the size of a person's head; this had been scientifically established by his countryman Paul Broca and confirmed, Binet declared, "by all methodical investigators, without exception."[46] But Binet was a conscientious scientist, and in time he not only revised his ideas about how intelligence could be measured, but discovered and wrote honestly about his unconscious tendency to be influenced by his own preconceptions—to increase the measurement of the heads of intelligent subjects and decrease the measurement of unintelligent ones. He abandoned head-measuring in favor of a new approach in which children were asked to perform intellectual tasks. The result, which eventually became the "intelligence quotient," scored the subject's performance as the "mental age" and compared that to the chronological age.

Binet never believed that his tests measured inherent intelligence; he saw them as a tool for discovering children who needed special education. But when intelligence testing emigrated to the United States, it took on a new identity. Henry Goddard, the historian of the Kallikak family, was the first American to employ such tests. Goddard had no doubt that intelligence was a genetic trait: "a unit character and transmitted in true Mendelian fashion."[47]

Intelligence testing was carried forward by American pioneers: Lewis M. Terman developed the Stanford-Binet test; Robert M. Yerkes sold the U.S. Army on the idea of intelligence testing and ran 1.75 million recruits through tests during World War I. The results confirmed the expectations of the eugenicists: Soldiers of Anglo-Saxon descent were found to be more intelligent than soldiers of Mediterranean and Eastern European extraction, whites did better than blacks, and the overall mental age was shockingly low—indicating that the population as a whole was going down the drain because of immigration and interbreeding. The Army tests were a major influence on Congress' decision to adopt immigration quotas.

In England, where social prejudice followed class lines more than racial ones, and where there was no tide of foreign immigration to exacerbate national anxieties, intelligence testing had a different but still significant social impact. Sir Cyril Burt, for many years dean of British psychologists, believed it to be "incontestable" that intelligence was "a general factor entering into every kind of cognitive process," and that this general factor depended largely "on the individual's genetic constitution."[48] Burt's research with pairs of twins who had grown up apart from one another appeared to demonstrate conclusively that genetic destiny was a far more important force than the conditions under which they were raised and educated— nature over nurture. Burt's work and that of others of similar persuasions formed the basis for the "eleven-plus" examinations which tested schoolchildren and determined whether they would proceed onward and upward through the "grammar school" system to a university education or be shunted off into another set of schools which would prepare them for less auspicious futures at lower social levels.

Thousands of lives were affected by intelligence testing— thousands of people denied entry into the United States (or deported from Ellis Island after being identified as feebleminded); thousands of British boys and girls sorted out and branded as gifted, ordinary, or inferior. These public policies were not based on any scientific certainty. They may not have been based on falsehood, but their premises were, to say the least, subject to question.

IQ testing rests on a very shaky foundation. It has never been proved that there is a single entity called intelligence, and there are other serious problems: the notorious tendency of intelligence tests to be bound to a certain cultural heritage (in the World War I Army tests, for example, recruits, many of them new immigrants, were asked questions about American brand names and baseball players); the dubious mathematical assumptions and occasional fudging of data necessary to obtain a single measure of intelligence; the terrifying conditions under which they have sometimes been administered. Liberals protest against viewing intelligence as an inborn quality rather than as something capable of being remedied by improved social conditions, and contend that high IQ scores reflect environmental and educational advantages as much as inherent capability.

The most serious setback of all to the scientific solidity of the IQ/hereditarian position was the news that Burt's famous research on pairs of identical twins raised apart was fraudulent, as was some of his other work—including IQ correlations between close relatives and data on declining levels of intelligence in Britain.[49]

Such critiques and revelations do not discredit the whole enterprise of intelligence testing or the case for hereditary intelligence—which has considerably more going for it than Sir Cyril's research. They do, however, demonstrate vividly that we have not yet achieved any "objective" measurement of human superiority; and without one, all programs for breeding superior people remain matters of personal opinion. Society cannot find a consensus for the kind of eugenic policies that Galton and his followers yearned for, and neither can it find a basis for preventing a group with the means to do so from setting up a sperm or embryo bank and bringing into the world thousands of offspring of some alleged genius.

It is easier to establish with some certainty—and with hope of achieving social consensus—the presence of genetic defect. Yet even on the negative side there are great possibilities of error.

The pronouncements of the early eugenicists about feeblemindedness, criminality, and the supposed characterological shortcomings of people of various ethnic backgrounds were little more than the biases of the time decorated with a thin veneer of science. A few decades farther along, the discovery of a high prevalance of an extra Y chromosome in male inmates of an institution for the criminally insane led to a premature declaration that science had discovered the very gene for criminality. A number of scientists rushed into print with cries of Eureka and data purporting to describe these genetic villains: They were tall and aggressive, and punishment could not deter them.[50] The public was informed (incorrectly, it turned out later) that mass murderer Richard Speck possessed the dread Y chromosome. Then the inevitable second round of studies came along, and unveiled a far murkier picture: There was indeed some statistical correlation between the XYY pattern and incarceration, but it was very hard to say why. No gene for altriusm, no gene for criminality either.

Even the category of single-gene defects—where matters are much more clearly defined—refuses to yield simple answers. Genetic screening and counseling can provide reliable state-of-the-art information—but much of it still comes in the form of probabilities rather than certainties. In regard to PKU, foremost among the defects believed to be detectable through genetic screening, the history has been far from perfect: children with PKU not detected, children without it incorrectly identified and placed on the prescribed diet.[51]

In other screening methods, such as prenatal amniocentesis to detect Down's syndrome, the findings are now more reliable but the parents still face a difficult choice; science does not print out the answer. Children with Down's syndrome are not all of a kind—some have IQ scores in the 20-40 range and others have scores as high as 80; there is much that can be done to increase their abilities and help them lead satisfying lives. The decision to abort may be the wisest, but it is not one that can be made automatically. It is a human choice in which values, hopes, feelings, and religious beliefs are as important as data.

As genetic screening and counseling touch more private lives, more and more people are discovering that the information they are given is not a clear picture of some small "thing" that "causes" a specific disorder, but rather a glimpse of a set of probabilities. The information encoded in the genes does not stamp out a human being like an item off the assembly line, but only sets in motion a line of interactions with the environment—with ecosystems, with workplaces and polluted cities, with society.

Yet the information is there, and so is the information *about* information which is the stock in trade of that perplexing new feedback loop in human life, genetic screening. We have more information in our lives and more is on the way; the task at hand is to understand what we know.

The Numbers Game: Malthus v. Pangloss

POPULATION was the first evolutionary-governance issue, and remains the predominant one. It forces us to come to terms with our own peculiar position in the biosphere; it reveals both our ability to transcend the limits set by nature upon other species, and our inability to avoid the consequences.

The first priests of progress envisioned a future of ever-increasing freedom and abundance, but feared that such utopian dreams might never be realized in a world with too many people. Condorcet and Godwin considered the matter and persuaded themselves it was not such a great danger after all—but then the Reverend Malthus joined in with a formulation that not only monopolized the con-

[193]

versation for centuries, but provided Charles Darwin with a critical piece of his theory of evolution.

Malthus' famous essay was about biology and politics: about what he perceived as an inevitable increase of human numbers beyond food supplies, and about whether public assistance to the poor might not make matters worse by encouraging them to marry and multiply.[52]

Darwin seized upon Malthus' observation that human beings tended to reproduce in greater numbers than were needed to keep population stable, so that—in the absence of checks such as war or plague—population would double and redouble. As Darwin saw it, the principle of over-reproduction was virtually universal in nature and led to constant evolutionary change as less fit offspring were eliminated by forces in the environment and the fitter reproduced. It was clear to all the participants in this dialogue that the human species had gained a degree of control over its own survival unlike anything to be found elsewhere in the world; this was apparent two centuries ago, well before iron lungs, dialysis machines, and genetically-engineered insulin.

Human population does not increase at a simple geometrical rate, but it does show a pattern of exponential growth—increasing rate of increase. Its upward-sweeping curve has become one of the familiar icons of our time.

Paul Ehrlich, who brought Malthusian misgivings into modern consciousness with his book *The Population Bomb,* described exponential growth in terms of doubling time: The human population, he said, had taken probably a million years to double before 8000 B.C.—but was doubling about every 1000 years by the mid-seventeenth century, every 200 years by Darwin's time, and at present every 35 years. He pointed out that if growth were to continue at the current rate for about 900 years, there would be some sixty million billion people, about 100 of us for every square yard of the Earth's surface—land and sea.[53]

After nearly twenty controversy-ridden years, the basic outlines of Ehrlich's argument still hold up. They are (1) that human numbers have been escalating as a function of our increasing ability to manipulate the conditions of survival, (2) that the present rate of growth cannot continue, and that (3) we will have to learn how to intervene in a different way—to control population growth—in order to avoid a disastrous crunch between our population and the living infrastructure that supports it.

It became clear in the neo-Malthusian years of the late 1960s and early 1970s, that more was involved than food supplies. In some countries the doubling time was less than 20 years, and national economies would have to provide twice as many jobs, twice as many houses, twice as many schools, merely to maintain current levels of misery.

People who for various reasons did not want to accept any part of the contemporary population dialogue—either the description of the situation or the prescribed remedies—have tried very hard to portray it as a simple replay of Malthusianism. This is a good thing to do if you are trying to win points for your debating team, because Malthus was wrong. Population does not always increase geometrically, and food supply does not necessarily increase arithmetically—and, anyway, that is only a part of the issue. The population question goes far beyond food, literally touches every corner of the global ecosystem: The consequences of overpopulation include pollution, extinction of species, land erosion and genetic erosion, overuse of resources, massive migrations, and the growth of immense urban slums with millions of people living in abject hopelessness.

In the score of years since population re-asserted its claim as the salient biological-political question—the great disturber of our dreams of progress—enormous change has taken place. Enormous change, and at the same time enormous resistance to change. The optimist can find ample evidence that we are indeed capable of responding to information, altering course, dealing constructively and creatively with the challenges of evolutionary governance. The pessimist can find ample reason to believe we are at best clever primates, irrational and self-destructive, bound to a primitive consciousness that takes the world's well-being to be measurable by how many of us there are in it.

A lot has happened. In 1974, national representatives came together in an historic gathering: Organized by the UN, the world poulation conference at Bucharest was the first attempt of governments to look at human pop-ulation as a whole and to consider cooperative measures for dealing with it. The subject was new to most of the delegates; most countries had population policies of the sort that assumed higher population to be a sign of greater national strength. The people who were worried about *over*population seemed to come from the developed coun-tries; Third World representatives were deeply suspicious about the enthusiasm of well-fed white people for reducing populations among the poor and colored.

But the delegates listened to the data on population growth and what it meant, and out of the conference came a "World Population Plan of Action." The decade that followed brought new attitudes and practices, one of the most dramatic transitions in the recorded history of human evolution. In five years, Mexico's annual population growth went down by a third, from 3.4 percent to 2.3 percent. Other countries—among them Columbia, Costa Rica, Indonesia, Singapore, Sri Lanka, Thailand, and Zimbabwe—achieved striking reductions in growth rates.[54] In China, where Chairman Mao had once equated population growth with progress, the government re-thought its position, decided on a policy of two children per family, took a look at the projections on that, and re-thought again; the most ambitious growth-reduction policy ever, one child per family, became the goal of the world's most-populated nation.[55] African nations, once equally pronatalist, agreed in the "Kilimanjaro Declaration" of 1984 to provide free or subsidized family-planning services.[56]

However, the course of human events usually marches in at least two directions at the same time; the global population initiative set in motion a phalanx of counter-moves. The Roman Catholic church, alarmed by the population-control policies of some Catholic countries and the statistics on use of contraceptives by Catholics (nearly 80 percent in the United States), issued a "Charter on Family Rights" opposing birth control programs.[57] Other religious opposition emerged: Fundamentalist Protestantism is opposed to family planning, and so is fundamentalist Islam.

In the United States, which had been the major supporter of family-planning activities worldwide, a well-financed opposition movement surfaced. Its theoretician was Julian Simon, an economist whose earlier field of specialization had been mail-order business and who now came forth with a theory—much like that of the early Mao—which equated more people with more prosperity. Simon contends that "The standard of living has risen along with the size of the world's population since the beginning of recorded time," and is convinced that the two will continue onward and upward together.[58] Simon's thesis appealed mightily to conservative, fundamentalist, and anti-environmentalist groups who, having found so many of the proposed solutions to overpopulation unpalatable, were receptive to the argument that there was no problem. He became the resident expert on population for the conservative Heritage Foundation and co-edited a book with Herman Kahn, our century's Condorcet and salesman for the contemporary version of the belief that nothing will stand in the way of progress.

Although the main cadre of anti-population control activism is made up of right-wing political forces—conservative Catholics, Bible Belt protestants, Julian Simon and his colleagues at the Heritage Foundation—population does not fit into a simple left-right categorization and never has. It is not an Industrial Revolution question but a fundamental issue of human evolution, older than the Industrial Revolution and taking on new urgency in the Biological Revolution as science—working both sides of the street—produces new ways of increasing population growth and new ways of reducing it. There are right-wing anti-population control forces, conservatives who see overpopulation as likely to increase the possibility of Communist revolution in Third World countries, Catholic countries with family-planning programs and legal abortion, old-school Marxists opposed to population control, and endless further variations.

But there is a fundamental polarization between those who favor population control policies and those who oppose them. The contending forces are bitterly drawing the battle lines, and a major worldwide conflict is already in motion. The great majority of people have not chosen to enlist on either side, have not quite accepted the warnings of dire global effects from overpopulation, nor bought the opposing argument that the 6.1 billion people forecast for 1999 is the best of all possible worlds.

Population is an old problem and a new one, and painfully difficult to comprehend. It is a quintessentially information-era kind of problem: It comes to most of us in the Western world in the form of data and interpretations of data.

Information comes in, and is often misunderstood. The average American believes that overpopulation is a problem, but reads in the newspaper of falling birth rates and is reassured—does not grasp the image of millions of people moving into the childbearing years, the astonishing reality of 150 people being added to the world per minute, 9000 an hour, 216,000 per day, about 80 million a year.[59] Something is happening that has not happened before; we have never added such numbers of people to the web of the planet's life, and nobody on any side of the dialogue knows what consequences it will produce.

Biology, Ecology and Social Contracts

In 1968, the year *The Population Bomb* was published, another biologist, Garrett Hardin, wrote an essay entitled "The Tragedy of the Commons." Hardin's essay was in part a parable, about what happens to a peaceful open pasture when the herds belonging to the various people who use it grow beyond the carrying capacity of the land. It was also a political tract with an explosive argument.

Only a year earlier some thirty nations had agreed: "The Universal Declaration of Human Rights describes the family as the natural and fundamental unit of society. It follows that any choice and decision with regard to the size of the family must irrevocably rest with the family itself, and cannot be made by anyone else."[60] That had expressed the very essence of political respectability, and seemed invulnerable to any challenge from left or right. Hardin challenged it—said that the biological conditions had been changed by overpopulation, and that it was time for the governments of the world to adopt policies, coercive ones if necessary, to get people to have fewer children.

The appearance of such a political tract and its acceptance by many people (it quickly became a staple of environmental literature) are all parts of the learning process which the contemporary population dialogue has set in motion. It would have been unthinkable a few centuries earlier for anyone to propose that the size of a family in one part of the world somehow mattered to people in another part of the world; there would have been no information available to form the basis for such an idea, no concept of global ecological impacts for it to make a difference, and no dependable methods and materials of birth control to create a reasonable expectation that people could plan their family size without resorting to celibacy or infanticide.

Regardless of what position you may take on the controversial issues that the population activists raise, there is a profound significance in the very appearance of such an issue. Suddenly we are confronted with an image of the global commons, and with data about human population and the patterns of its growth. Such images train our vision; we see the arena of political interaction in a global context—and there is no retreating from such an expansion of the field of view.

All our laws and constitutions and political philosophies are descended from parables about social interaction, framed by images of the environments in which human beings relate, shaped by information about how one person's action impacts upon another life. If you look closely at the work of any of the master political philosophers, be it Aristotle with the polis or Rousseau with the state of nature, you can begin to discern the dimensions of the frame—and see that it is considerably less than global. Human beings played out their lives and made their political demands upon one another in relatively cozy spaces.

Now, suddenly, the frame expands: It matters in one country if industries in another produce acid rain. If one nation is overpopulated it matters to people in adjoining countries from which the overpopulated country's people must obtain firewood and food and into which refugees will inevitably migrate. And, since population movement is global and a global communications network flashes to comfortable Americans the news of the latest famine in some eroded Third World nation, it matters around the world.

Social contracts emerge out of contact, the polis grows out of perceived interdependence. For the first time in human history, people find it reasonable to ask other people to limit the size of their families. The population control issue is an attempt to negotiate a new global social contract, in which all people accept membership in one commons. But it is an explosive business in many ways: The debate is not merely about numbers but also about consumption of resources; Paul Ehrlich always insisted that the most overpopulated nation of all was the United States, because of its high consumption of resources and energy per person. Racism and nationalism are never far in the background; the current anxiety in many European countries about their falling birthrates partakes generously of both. Also, the pattern of world migration—from the Third World to the relatively uncrowded spaces of Europe and North America—suggests that yet another demand is being made on the global commons: the demand for the right to move freely to places where there is the possibility of employment or land.

Rafael M. Salas, head of the United Nations' Fund for Population Activities, has said that the dominant metaphor for the population crisis should be not a "population bomb" but a "population wave," gathering strength and momentum as it sweeps through the world. The wave is a useful image, certainly superior to descriptions of population as a "problem" that can somehow be "solved". The problem will not be solved, the crisis will not be averted; it is already here. Governments and international organizations and private individuals can modify the size of the wave, but not dispel it. It will roll through history until, probably, sometime in the next century, total human numbers begin to decline for the first time; for the first time in the course of Earth's evolution, a species will have achieved the will and the ability to limit its own size.

Achieving the will is largely a political matter, and is the central subject of the huge global dialogue that is now in progress, as people and governments consider the information, consult their beliefs and values, and make decisions. The dialogue is proceeding rapidly, although with the backlashes and confusions that inevitably attend social change. The ability is more in the realm of science, where things are moving very rapidly indeed. Most of the birth control methods now in use are of fairly recent origin, and new developments are on the way. They will, of course, affect the political equation; it seems quite likely, for example, that if dependable abortifacient suppositories become available—thereby enabling a woman to make the decision about abortion entirely her own—it will become extremely difficult for any government to enforce any law against abortion. One of the curious developments of our time is that, while matters of human reproduction become more politicized by information about global and evolutionary impacts, they become more privatized by scientific developments which enable the individual to make more choices about his or her own biological life.

Population activists are not enthusiastic about the boom in new reproductive technologies, *in vitro* fertilization and the rest of the growing package, but I suspect that in the long run they have little to fear from this quarter. It is clear already that when women have control over their reproductive lives and access to other roles besides that of mother, they do not choose to have great numbers of children. The change that is taking place is an alteration in the basic conditions of human life, a shift toward increasing intentionality and choice, and it enables people to transcend the biological destiny that Malthus and Darwin discussed.

As reproduction becomes increasingly a matter of choice it will be shaped by many factors including public policy and social pressure—factors that will reflect prevailing beliefs about whether overpopulation is or is not a threat to the human future—and inevitably eugenic considerations will also play a part. We know that they do already, in fact, as more people make reproductive decisions on the basis of information about their genetic makeup.

Eugenics never went away. Quite the contrary: Now we are all eugenicists, concerned about improvement or deterioration of the species and, furthermore, able to make decisions about it. And all governments, whether they know it or not, have eugenics policies. They have one kind of policy if they sponsor genetic screening and family planning programs, another kind if they outlaw abortion and require doctors to make superhuman efforts to save babies born with serious defects.

Most eugenics policies are unacknowledged ones, of course, and most governments probably have different policies that work in opposite directions. But this state of innocence will not be allowed to continue, as more becomes known about human genetics and more methods of conception and birth control become available to more people. Every government will be obliged to articulate its population and evolution policies, and people will make reproductive decisions of different kinds and for different reasons than anything known to past generations.

People often complain of the intrusion of government into private life in regard to these matters, and that is a valid concern; the first round of eugenics policies showed vividly the threat of violation of civil rights by misinformed technocrats bent on improving the species. But life, unfortunately, is not as private as it used to be: Population growth, sperm banks, frozen embryos, genetic screening, and many other aspects of the contemporary human biological situation take private life into the domain of political and social interaction. Yet at the same time, individual options—and, in a sense, personal freedom—increase.

As we begin to perceive the outlines of our political future, the most attractive prospect that presents itself to the liberal imagination is one in which the government's role is that of facilitator and provider of information— about world population, about genetic defects, about birth control—and the locus of decision-making is at the individual level. It won't ever be that neat, of course, but even to sketch out such a possibility gives us a reminder of the remarkable extent to which the new issues of biopolitics erode the old boundary between public and private life and turn our most personal acts into acts of participation in the polis. When governance is seen in a biological context there are still inequities, but there are no nonparticipants.[61]

It is tempting to want to withdraw from such engagement, to declare that neither governments nor individuals have the right to intervene in the biological actions of the human organism, that to do so is to play God. But we know too much now to find our way back to that Eden. It becomes increasingly clear that as we take responsibility for our reproductive lives, our obligations to the global commons and to the future, we are not playing God but being human.

[6]

The Rights of
Living Things

THE POLIS has always been a community of human beings, and in actual practice has rarely even been very inclusive about that: All states have excluded from full citizenship some or most of the people over whom they claimed dominion. The great majority of people have occupied inferior and in some cases scarcely human status in their societies. Classical Athens, that early model of democracy, gave full rights of citizenship to only about one-tenth of its population of 400,000 or so. The remainder were women, children, foreigners and slaves.

Modern civilization has seen a tumultuous sequence of moves to bring new groups of people into equal citizenship: abolition of slavery and serfdom, elimination of property qualifications to vote, women's suffrage. These have been disturbing enough—seen by many as hideously radical extremism—but at least they have had to do with extending rights to human beings. Indeed, when Mary Shelley wrote an early feminist essay entitled *A Vindication of the Rights of Women*, somebody else wrote a parody of it entitled *A Vindication of the Rights of Brutes*, intended to prove that if the same arguments could be applied to animals they were for that reason out of the question.[1]

But now in many ways people are seeking to extend the boundaries of the polis beyond what has for so long seemed to be its obvious limits, the collectivity of living human beings. Conservationists insist that the interests of generations yet unborn must be part of current decision-making. Anti-abortion crusaders champion the rights of the fetus and seek legal status for the cells in a petri dish that have the potential to become human beings. And another movement—actually a many-sided surge of movements—is now fighting for the rights of non-human entities that were merely parts of the furniture in the polis that Aristotle saw when he first deliberated about the nature of the political animal.

The animal rights movement has more legitimacy than it had in Mary Shelley's day, but it is still not quite accepted as a serious political movement. The time has come to take it seriously, as a principled attempt to redefine some of our most basic concepts about the nature of political rights and obligations.

Furthermore, its emergence as a political force at this time is not an accident, but the reflection of basic changes in the conditions of our biological existence—changes which, although unknown and unseen by most human beings, have transformed the nature of our relationship to the animals upon whom our lives depend.

Today's Holocaust

IN *The Space Merchants*, a classic science-fiction novel of the 1950s, there is a monstrosity called Chicken Little: a gigantic tissue culture, so huge that human beings can move through tunnels inside it. It absorbs nutrients and endlessly grows more flesh which is trimmed from its sides by knife-wielding laborers and sold as food.[2]

Chicken Little remains science fiction, not fact, but there is an historical process at work—a transformation of food production into something less like farming, more like industry—that the novel foreshadowed. Dairy cattle, meat animals, and egg-laying chickens live lives of strange captivity in which they are merely elements in a mechanized system that converts animal feed into protein for human consumption.

These modern factory farms are not as spectacular as the scene in *The Space Merchants*, but the reality of them is far more hideous in terms of the amount of suffering involved. Chicken Little was a brainless mountain of tissue; the animal cogs in present-day food-producing machines are conscious products of evolution, some of them highly intelligent, all of them capable of feeling pain—which they do throughout their lifetimes.

About 95 percent of the eggs consumed in the United States come from "battery hens" whose lives are spent in cramped and crowded wire cages where each hen has less than one square foot of space to herself.[3] The battery cages deliver food, collect eggs, and carry away feces. The hens often exhibit insane and destructive behavior, called "vices": They try to peck one another to death, and the routine precaution against this is to cut off their beaks; de-beaking—a painful mutilation—leaves the hen capable of feeding but incapable of doing any damage to herself or to her neighbors.

There are other miseries. Normally hens lay eggs in cycles then stop laying to moult; in the battery cage system, premature moulting is forced by depriving the hen of water for three or four days and of food for another seven to ten. This produces more eggs, but the chickens commonly develop bone problems from the calcium loss. When eggs are hatched the chicks are culled. Females and a few males are retained, and the remaining males are disposed of in various ways: One method is to throw them into plastic garbage bags which are then crushed.

Calves for premium veal are raised in similar circumstances. They are confined, for the 16 or so weeks that they live, in darkened isolation in pens too small to permit turning around. Deprived of water in order to keep their thirst high, they consume large quantities of a low-iron milk substitute which induces a state of borderline anemia; this gives their meat the pale color prized in gourmet restaurants.

Pigs are rarely to be found any more wallowing about in sloppy contentment in pastures and pig pens; about 85 percent of hogs raised in the United States are now tightly confined in nursery cages for piglets, in gestation crates for pregnant sows, or in automated "bacon bins" which hold 500 animals and can be tended by one man.[4] Like other confined animals they develop vices, most commonly a tendency to bite one another's tails; this is dealt with by cutting their tails off. Pigs, the most intelligent of domestic animals, are also susceptible to a neurosis, known in the trade as "porcine stress syndrome." It produces a variety of physical and behavioral symptoms, and occasionally results in sudden death.

These tribulations of automated food production can be costly to the farmer, but on the whole the new methods are productive and profitable—which is of course their reason for being. The change that has been taking place in the past decades—and few urban readers are likely to be aware of how dramatic the change has been, how rapidly it is still unfolding—is essentially an afterthought of the Industrial Revolution. Its methods, its innovative spirit, its basic willingness to subordinate all values to those of the marketplace, are those of early industry; and the animals of the factory farms are the modern counterparts of the miserable wage slaves of the eighteenth century. Industry and agriculture, so long separate fields of human endeavor, are no longer distinguishable from one another. The merger is hastened along by many forces, among them the needs of growing urban populations, the cost and scarcity of land, the increase of agribusiness and absentee ownership, the promotional activity of feed and equipment suppliers, the policies of agriculture departments and government-funded research in the universities. All these conspire to create a new kind of food production.

Agriculture has never been kind to animals. There is a long history of monstrosities like the forced stuffing of geese to produce *pâté de foie gras,* and I saw during my own cattle-ranch youth that there was plenty of cruelty in the cowboy life so dear to American folklore. I remember well the branding irons glowing red in the wood fire, and the smell of burning hair and flesh; I know what it is like to spend long hot afternoons in a dusty corral castrating calves with a pocket knife. Yet even a person who is without illusions about agriculture as it was can recognize clearly—perhaps even more clearly—that it is becoming something far different.

Another facet of animal rights is the use of animals in experimentation. Modern science is a prodigious consumer of animal life: dogs and cats, rabbits, farm animals, primates, reptiles, birds, frogs, rats and mice. An Office of

Technology Assessment report estimates 17 to 22 million animals now used annually in the U. S. including 12 to 15 million rats and mice.[5] Some animal rights spokesmen claim the total number is closer to 100 million.[6]

Supplying this demand is another business, as strange in its way as the factory farms. Charles River Breeding Laboratories, Inc., known as "the General Motors of animal breeding," is a large operation which owns two primate breeding islands, has subsidiaries in several countries, and produces some 14 million animals a year for the laboratories. Its catalog features such specialties as rats that are highly susceptible to arthritis and others guaranteed to develop high blood pressure at the age of six weeks.[7] Many smaller organizations ply the same trade, as do importers legal and illegal, and many cat and dog pounds.

The animals are dissected by students in biology classes; operated upon to try out surgical procedures; given diseases and drugs; exposed to chemicals intended for human use in foods and household products; given cancers and possible treatments for it; subjected to mock automobile accidents; implanted with electrodes and run through psychological tests; shot, bombed, and napalmed in military weapons testing centers. Few of the uses are pleasant to the animals, and some are outright torture, either physical or mental, experiments in which the agony of the animal is not an unfortunate by-product of the work, but its purpose.

For example, scientists at the Primate Research Center of the University of Wisconsin observed the behavior of female monkeys that had been driven insane by torture and then made pregnant. A mother, they noted, would sometimes crush her infant's skull with her teeth; another would smash her infant's face against the floor and rub it back and forth.[8] Such experiments were supposed to shed some light upon human psychosis and, presumably, lessen the suffering in the world.

The common justification for such experimentation is that it saves human lives. That is true of a small fraction of it. Most of it is academic busywork which produces no results at all or, in the case of the psychological experiments, conclusions of stunning banality.

The arguments about trends in agriculture and laboratory experimentation, pro and con, sometimes obscure an important evolutionary point—which is that the upward human progress in the present century is matched by a deterioration in the quality of life for the rest of creation. The number of animals used in laboratory experimentation has increased enormously, and a great portion of that use involves either pain inflicted incidentally to the main purpose of the research, or pain inflicted deliberately and with a high degree of scientific knowledge of how to go about making living creatures suffer. With such a massive increase of misery taking place in a world whose people fancy themselves to be becoming more civilized, it was inevitable that some sort of an opposition movement would emerge.

The Movement

IN THE MIDST of a glittering event at the Shubert Theatre in New York city, where stars and socialites had gathered for a musical revue and fur show to benefit the city's museum, a couple of young demonstrators stood up and began shouting slogans such as: "No cruelty to animals!" and "Furriers are murderers!" Just before they were thrown out, they unrolled an eight-foot long banner which proclaimed: REAL PEOPLE WEAR FAKE FURS. Later, outside, a well-dressed young man approached one of them and said: "I just want you to know that you ruined a wonderful evening." The demonstator replied that that had been exactly the point.[9]

At the University of Pennsylvania, masked members of an organization called the Animal Liberation Front broke into a laboratory where primates were used in head-injury research and stole videotapes of the experiments. The tapes, which showed the work in gruesome detail and also recorded the joking comments of the experimenters, were called the "Watergate tapes of the animal rights movement."[10]

The animal liberation movement arises in a society which, whatever its innocence about evolutionary politics, is familiar with protest. So, although the movement's content is new, its methods are familiar: civil disobedience, lobbying, lawsuits, public education programs, demonstrations. It is represented by a bumper crop of new organizations, a hard core of old ones beginning to feel a bit threatened by the rowdy upstarts, and a brigade of theoreticians to argue its moral case.

A recent issue of a guide to the alternative press contains a list of animal rights periodicals: Among them are *The Animal's Agenda*, *Flesh and Blood*, *Liberator*, *One World*, and *Outcry*. Among the organizations they represent: Animal Rights Network, Compassion in World Farming, International Primate Protection League, British Union for the Abolition of Vivisection, People for the Ethical Treatment of Animals, and Trans-Species Unlimited.[11] There is also an Animal Legal Defense Fund that battles for animal rights in the courts.

The energies of the newer organizations tend to go into protests and other actions designed to raise public awareness as dramatically as possible, and some of them have been notably successful. One was the campaign against the "Draize test," a method of testing the toxicity of cosmetics, detergents, oven cleaners and similar products by dropping solutions of them into the eyes of rabbits. A lone activist in New York started a campaign against the Draize test in 1979, and by the end of that year over 400 animal welfare organizations had joined in. After a couple of years of media advertisements and protest actions aimed at the cosmetics industry and government agencies, the protestors had this to show for their efforts:

(1) The Revlon Corporation made a $750,000 grant to Rockefeller University for study of alternative tests.
(2) A cosmetics trade association organized a Draize test workshop and pledged $1 million for research on alternatives.
(3) Other companies—Avon, Estee Lauder, Bristol-Meyers, Chanel, Mary Kay and Max Factor—also pledged research funds.
(4) A center for alternatives to animal testing was established at Johns Hopkins University.
(5) The Food and Drug Administration committed funds for similar research.
(6) A resolution was introduced in Congress instructing all federal agencies that use the Draize test to develop other approaches.[12]

Another landmark victory for the movement was the conviction of Dr. Edward Taub, chief scientist at the Institute for Behavioral Research in Silver Spring, Maryland, on charges of cruelty to animals. Taub's work involved deadening the limbs of monkeys by severing nerves at the spinal cord, but that was not the issue: He was put on trial for failing to provide the animals with the minimal care required by law. The charges against Taub were the result of undercover work by Alex Pacheco, a young animal rights activist who had gone to work in the lab. Pacheco found monkeys confined in damaged cages, some with open and untreated wounds, others that had chewed fingers off or dug holes in their chests. He began making notes and taking photographs and took his information to the police, who came to the laboratory with a search and seizure warrant; the police took documents and 17 of the monkeys, and charged Taub and an assistant with cruelty to animals.[13]

The controversy surrounding Taub and Pacheco and the "Silver Spring 17," as the monkeys became known, went far beyond the criminal charges, on which Taub was found guilty and fined. The National Institute of Health suspended its $115,000 grant to Taub; Department of Agriculture officials were reprimanded for their failure to enforce the federal Animal Welfare Act, which regulates the care and keeping of laboratory animals; and some scientists expressed their resentment of such attacks on research. A state appeals court later overturned Taub's conviction on grounds that the state anti-cruelty laws did not apply to federally-funded research—but by that time Taub's laboratory was closed and an animal rights group was suing for custody of the monkeys, hoping to be able to place them in one of the many sanctuaries for "liberated" laboratory animals that are now in operation. Researchers across the country had begun to change their practices in regard to the treatment of laboratory animals and, although the case had nothing to do with animal experimentation itself, the public had developed a bit more awareness that the life of a laboratory animal is not a happy one.

[215]

The animal rights activists are also interested in hunting. The Committee to Abolish Sport Hunting, which the National Rifle Association calls "one of the most dangerous and aggressive organizations in the United States," has challenged the formidable hunting establishment both in the courts and in protest actions. Another organization, Friends of Animals, hands out instructions for people who want to take part in "hunt sabotage":

> Get into the woods the day before hunting season. Try to drive wildlife away. Stroll about with a loud radio. . . . If hunters use dogs in your area, try to get hold of a female dog in heat and lead her, on a leash, through an area that is heavily hunted. Male dogs in the hunter's pack will "get wind" of the female and lose their enthusiasm for chasing rabbits or other hunted animals. . . . If you have a portable tape recorder, buy a cassette recording of wolf howls. Play this in the woods a few times in the days before hunting season.[14]

The anti-hunting campaign has not been widely publicized, but it is potentially a major issue of evolutionary governance because—in the United States and many other countries—much of the management of ecosystems is carried out by agencies whose sole clients are hunters and fishermen. To benefit the sportsmen, rivers and lakes are stocked with fish, animals are imported and bred, predators are controlled and other uses regulated. The animal rights people challenge this management rationale at every turn: They question the "cropping" whereby authorities reduce populations of game animals by unleashing hunters, question the time-honored practice of financing fish and game agencies with license fees, and on the whole push toward

[216]

a complete rethinking of the principles according to which governments determine the numbers and types of animals that shall be permitted to exist on public lands.

There are many other fields of animal rights activity: Greenpeace on the seas harassing the whalers, local activists crusading for drug injection instead of suffocation as a method of euthanasia for pound animals, lawyers working on animal rights cases, veterinarians being taught animal rights issues as part of their professional education. The movement is rapidly gaining converts, and also making powerful political enemies—many research scientists, farmers, farm equipment manufacturers, professional fishermen, hunters, and the NRA. It is also revealing occasional excesses in its search for a kind of moral purity that has never been clearly defined and has produced serious internal conflicts between the newcomers and the older organizations. A publication of Trans-Species Unlimited charges:

> The traditional animal welfare/humane movement has hypocritically focused almost all of its attention on domestic animal issues, while ignoring more pervasive, *institutionalized* abuses which occur daily but pass largely unnoticed by the general public. Moreover, in their preference for domestic animals many of these groups are guilty of speciesism, and in some cases have even supported practices which are clearly exploitative of animals, and/or contribute to animal suffering as a whole, e.g., the promotion of pet shows, cropping of dogs' ears and declawing of cats, and breeding of animals for pleasure or profit.[15]

The movement, then, is anything but monolithic. It has created not only a dialogue between the activists and the public, but heated and often acrimonious internal dispute.

Rights in Evolution

SOME ISSUES of evolutionary governance can be stated in terms of resources and material self-interest and discussed without getting too far into ethical territory—but the dialogue that the animal rights movement has opened up is inescapably a *moral* dialogue.

Politics is, just below its surface of ego, power and money, largely a process of moral growth anyway. This tends to make Americans uncomfortable, infatuated as we are with our folk religion of economics; we like to believe that all political outcomes are determined by "real" motives like greed, and we are faintly embarassed by any discussion of right and wrong that cannot be reduced to such terms.

Yet despite our national shyness about such matters, American history has been a chorus of sermons and a series of moral ordeals. We have struggled with racism and sexism, with military power and abortion, with prayer in school and capital punishment. And, although the going has been rough and progress fitful, there is no doubt that cultural values have changed tremendously over the short span of time that our history represents.

The animal rights movement is a public course in ethics, and it is an adventure in human evolution—a dominant species becoming reluctantly aware of its moral responsibility toward other forms of life. Animal rights is also, like so many of the other concerns of evolutionary governance, a religious question; the position one takes in relation to it reflect one's basic beliefs about the role the human species plays in the larger drama of the cosmos.

Consequently theologians are prominently involved, and on all sides there is much quoting from Genesis.

It is a moral debate long overdue, one in which the animals have a lot of ground to gain. The Bible gave them into human dominion, and the Catholic church has taught that they have no souls. Descartes placed them outside the category of thinking beings, classed them as a variety of machinery; and Kant, that great moral philosopher who spoke so forcefully against regarding a human being as a means to an end, saw animals as means, not ends in themselves. The prevailing view has been that they had neither feelings to be hurt nor any kind of moral intelligence.

Yet, despite this view, which has exiled animals from the network of rights and obligations that form human society, there is a long and bizarre history of animals having been tried and punished for crimes—not only in one or two whimsical instances, but in many places and over the centuries. Ecclesiastical and civil authorities have charged and convicted all kinds of beasts, from domestic animals to field mice and worms, of all kinds of crimes, from misdemeanors to murder. In one case a horde of locusts were excommunicated for destroying crops, a curious punishment for beings without souls. Animals have been punished by imprisonment, flogging, banishment (a Russian court exiled a goat to Siberia in the late seventeenth century), and frequently execution: A rooster was burned at the stake in Basel for witchcraft (he had laid an egg, allegedly in compact with Satan). A sow in France was hanged for murder (her piglets, accomplices in the deed, were pardoned). In Connecticut, several farm animals were sentenced to death by hanging for having taken part in sexual acts with the farmer, who was also hanged.[16]

Such incidents seem to reflect a profound ambivalence toward animals, a feeling that they were *not* mindless and soulless objects but somehow a part of the community of moral life. Yet such feelings, if they existed, were rarely articulated. It is hard to find much about the subject in the writings of philosophers prior to the nineteenth century. One exception was Jeremy Bentham: Bentham's utilitarian philosophy held that justice in society should be determined not on the basis of such fictions as "natural law", but on a calculus of pleasure and pain; his most famous principle is that of the "greatest happiness of the greatest number." In *Principles of Morals and Legislation*, published in 1789, Bentham speculated that the same calculus could be applied to nonhuman life:

> The day *may* come when the rest of the animal creation may acquire those rights which never could have been withholden from them but by the hand of tyranny. The French have already discovered that the blackness of the skin is no reason why a human being should be abandoned without redress to the caprice of a tormentor. It may one day come to be recognized that the number of the legs, the villosity of the skin, or the termination of the *os sacrum* are reasons equally insufficient for abandoning a sensitive being to the same fate. What else is it that should trace the insuperable line? Is it the faculty of reason, or perhaps the faculty of discourse? But a full-grown horse or dog is beyond comparison a more rational, as well as a more conversable animal, than an infant of a day or a week or even a month, old. But suppose they were otherwise, what would it avail? The question is not, Can they *reason*? nor Can they *talk*? but, Can they *suffer*?

There was much interest in this question during Darwin's time. His writings—especially *The Origin of Species*, *The Descent of Man*, and *The Expression of the Emotions in Man and Animals*—altered ideas about animal life, and he was himself an active supporter of the humane cause, especially concerned about vivisection, a subject which, he said, made him "sick with horror."[17]

Many forces were pushing the issue toward the surface in those years: publicity about vivisection, the evolution debate, the common spectacle of horses flogged in the streets, the bears and other animals tormented for the public's amusement, the hunts in which English gentlefolk entertained themselves with the spectacle of small animals being dismembered by dog packs. Such practices led to the formation in 1836 of the Royal Society for the Prevention of Cruelty to Animals (Darwin was a member), and in 1866 of the American society.

Many forces are converging again in our own time to form what looks like an entirely new phase of animal rights activism. Among those are the changes in agriculture and the increase in animal experimentation, the legacy of the civil-rights and liberation movements which have created a public sensitivity to matters of rights and equality, and the environmental movement with its concern about species extinction and the destruction of natural habitat. The growth of the new movement has also been greatly stimulated by a lively output of work from young political philosophers.

One of these is Peter Singer, an Australian, whose work is in the Benthamite utilitarian tradition. Let us look at a short passage from his *Animal Liberation* to see how he takes Bentham's ideas through a consideration of the question of whether or not animals are "sentient" into a dis-

cussion of "speciesism", a concept with a distinctly contemporary flavor:

> If a being suffers there can be no moral justification
> for refusing to take that suffering into consideration.
> No matter what the nature of the being, the principle
> of equality requires that its suffering be counted equally
> with the like of any other being. If a being is not capable
> of suffering, or of experiencing enjoyment or happiness,
> there is nothing to be taken into account. So the limit
> of sentience (using the term as a convenient if not strictly
> accurate shorthand for the capacity to suffer and/or
> experience enjoyment) is the only defensible boundary
> of concern for the interests of others. To mark this
> boundary by some other characteristic like intelligence
> or rationality would be to mark it in an arbitrary manner.
> Why not choose some other characteristic, like skin
> color?
> The racist violated the principle of equality by giving
> greater weight to the interests of members of his own
> race when there is a clash between their interests and
> the interests of those of another race. The sexist violates
> the principle of equality by favoring the interests of his
> own sex. Similarly the speciesist allows the interests of
> his own species to override the greater interests of
> members of other species. The pattern is identical in
> any case.[18]

I chose the above passage because it gives an excellent
summary of a central argument of the animal rights movement and also because it suggests, in its invocations of
racism and sexism, how much the animal rights movement
is informed by the movements that have gone before.

I should mention that the movement's philosophical foundations are not entirely to be found in Singer and the Benthamite school. Another of the leading animal rights philosophers, Tom Regan, an American, agrees that animals have rights but does not agree that the subject should be approached in utilitarian terms. He criticizes utilitarianism for the some of the same reasons many thinkers have criticized it over the years: (1) that it looks great from a distance, but under close scrutiny becomes very unclear as to how to talk precisely about anybody's pain and pleasure and (2) that it reduces the being to a mere receptacle of experiences with no inherent value of its own. Regan prefers to come at the subject from an entirely different direction, from the point of view of inherent worth and thus inherent moral rights. He argues that, "like us, animals have certain basic moral rights, including in particular the fundamental right to be treated with the respect that, as possessors of inherent value, they are due as a matter of strict justice." [19]

Equally able spokesmen have come forth to argue that the case for inherent animal rights is carelessly reasoned and generally overstated, and that animals can never be regarded as members of the moral community. Michael Allen Fox, a Canadian philosopher, writes:

It is because they are capable of long-range planning, anticipating consequences, choosing among alternative courses of action, taking responsibility, making and following rules, and the like that humans can engage in moral behavior, or behavior that affects others as well as themselves and that is subject to moral appraisal. . . . Thus it appears that a moral community is a social group composed of interacting autonomous beings where moral concepts and precepts can evolve and be understood.[20]

So it would not be safe to conclude that there is an emerging public consensus about admitting animals to membership in the polis, or even agreement within the animal-rights movement as to *why* it should occur. Yet, even while the argument rages, governments move unsteadily toward substantial changes in the legal status of nonhuman life forms.

Rights Into Law

THE POLIS which, as Aristotle saw it, transformed the worst of animals into the best, was a system of laws—norms or moral precepts codified into rules of behavior accepted and enforced by society. The laws protected personal property, legitimized and limited the powers of leaders, and defended individuals against physical violence from others. Through law, human beings moved into a new mode of social interaction, and did in truth become a different kind of animal.

Humans were thus constrained into more civilized behavior toward other humans—but the political animal did not become noticeably more civilized in its dealings with other animals. They were merely property—if domestic, usually the property of individuals and subject to the laws that regulated ownership and exchange; if wild, usually the property of the state or the monarch. In either case, whatever laws applied to them were concerned with the wants and needs of human beings alone. The few early societies that had laws protecting animals for the sake of the animals themselves were usually those in the Orient guided by a belief in reincarnation—meaning that they saw animals as past or future humans.

The well-being of animals (except as property) did not hold a high priority in Western societies, although there are some recorded instances of early laws against cruelty to animals. In North America, the first such law was passed by the Massachusetts Bay Colony in 1641.

The cause made rapid progress in the nineteenth century, spurred along by the founding of the English and American societies for the prevention of cruelty to animals. By 1866, twenty American states and territories had passed anti-cruelty laws, and in 1876 the British Parliament passed the Cruelty to Animals Act.

The United States now has a sizeable body of legislation dealing in one way or another with animals: the federal Animal Welfare Act; anti-cruelty laws in all 50 states; the Endangered Species Act; and various others including the Migratory Bird Treaty Act (which restricts hunting of migratory birds), the Wild, Free-Roaming Horse and Burro Act (which prohibits killing or capturing wild horses and burros), and the Marine Mammal Protection Act (which outlaws whaling and gives other protections to marine mammals within U.S. waters.[21]

From the point of view of some people this is more than enough; from the point of view of animal rights activists it is a thin legal structure which outlaws a few cruelties, legitimizes many others, and is inadequately enforced. In 1982, a group of organizations brought suit against the Department of Agriculture, seeking more vigorous enforcement of the Animal Welfare Act. In 1985, a General Accounting Office report sharply criticized DOA's enforcement.

There is also a growing body of animal protection legislation in other countries: laws against hunting or exporting primates in some African countries, an extensive system of animal welfare protection in India, an endangered species program in the Soviet Union. Most Western European countries are well ahead of the U.S.: Switzerland banned battery cages for laying hens by a national referendum in 1981, Denmark's Protection of Animals Act outlaws the use of animals in circuses, and West Germany's law requires anyone keeping an animal to "provide accomodation which takes account of its natural behavior." The last item comes close to some of the provisions in the "bill of rights" proposed by some activists, which would require that captive animals be able to move about and perform natural functions such as grooming themselves. The Council of Europe is probably more active in promoting animal rights than any other international governmental body in the world.[22]

Some animal rights activists apply themselves to the passage or enforcement of laws at the local and state level, while others have their eye on the global picture. The international front is in some ways the most critical, and the least productive of quick victories.

One important international agency is the International Whaling Commission, which was created in 1946 to provide for the "rational exploitation of whales under international control" and has gradually been transformed into a somewhat more conservation-minded organization attempting to maintain stable levels of whales and prevent extinction of species. The Commission, caught between the interests of sovereign whaling nations and the pressure of conservationists, is trying with less than pure success to make the transition from cautious resource pie-cutting to evolutionary governance. In 1982 the IWC voted to end commercial whaling for five years, from 1986 to 1990—a move that was opposed by some whaling nations and promised a ticklish period of international arm-twisting while the majority tries to persuade the minority to go along with the decision.

Another international agency, created more recently and immediately plunged into the thick of the genetic rapids, is the Convention on International Trade in Endangered Species. CITES is the only international barricade against the massive exploitation of flora and fauna around the world—an exploitation that is of interest to animal lovers because of the cruelty and loss of life involved in it, and to conservationists because it contributes to the extinction of species. CITES has undoubtedly reduced wildlife smuggling, but its enforcement, which relies on the commitment of member nations and the competence of customs officers, is extremely sporadic.

Clearly we have a long distance to travel before animal rights and species protection become central concerns of the world's governments—but the activists are aiming high. One international organization proclaimed a Universal Declaration of the Rights of Animals in 1978, and has hopes of having it adopted by the United Nations. (See pp. 230–231.)

The battle to gain legal status for animal rights proceeds at many levels, then, from the local to the global, and along several fronts: getting laws passed, getting them enforced, getting favorable interpretations in the courts.

One of the more interesting legal issues that has arisen in this context is the question of standing. Christopher Stone, a University of Southern California law professor, wrote a book some years ago arguing that nonhuman entities should be granted standing in the courts to defend their rights. He began his case with the observation that any movement seeking to confer rights onto some new entity seems strange or ludicrous at first to those who already hold rights, but that at the appropriate stage of cultural evolution the rights of new groups—women, children, or slaves, for example—become thinkable. He took the discussion well beyond animal rights, however. His book was entitled *Should Trees Have Standing*, and it contended that a variety of natural objects, including non-living ones, could reasonably be given legal protection against destruction without excessive strain on the present framework of jurisprudence: "It is no answer," he wrote, "to say that streams and forests cannot have standing because streams and forests cannot speak. Corporations cannot speak either; nor can states, estates, infants, in-competents, municipalities or universities. Lawyers speak for them, as they customarily do for the ordinary citizen with legal problems."[23]

Stone's argument soon achieved a certain amount of legal legitimacy by being quoted by Supreme Court Justice William O. Douglas in his dissenting opinion in *Sierra Club v. Morton*, one of the first cases under the Endangered Species Act. And if you look at the record of the case of *Palila v. Hawaii*, which came before a federal court in 1979, you will notice that the plaintiff is not a corporation or an infant or a university, but a bird that lives on the slopes of Mauna Kea on the island of Hawaii. The islands' native flora and fauna—those not extinct already—are mostly endangered; the palila's evolutionary complaint was that it was being forced to share its fragile habitat with herds of sheep and goats, descendants of animals brought by Europeans, and now running more or less wild. Actually, the sheep and goats were being maintained

[228]

by the state government for the benefit of hunters. The animals and hunters were destroying the palila's habitat, pushing it ever closer to extinction, and the bird, with the help of the Sierra Club and the Audubon Society, sued the state, charging that the destruction of habitat constituted an unlawful "taking" of an endangered species contrary to federal law. The palila won its case, and the state was required to remove the goats and sheep from the premises.[24]

The matter of giving standing to a species of bird turns out to be—as Stone had thought—not so great a departure from a more human-centered view of the concept. But it vividly illustrates evolutionary governance in action, survival of species being determined by human law. A species is endangered, as species often are, by something happening in its habitat as a result of human intervention: in this case, descendants of imported goats and sheep chewing through the local flora and being pursued by gun-toting hunters. The ecosystem has been modified, new species have been introduced and pose a threat to a native species of a kind unlike anything in nature, and the whole thing winds up in court. It is a kind of evolution that Darwin never thought about, and it is the kind we will become familiar with in the years ahead.

The Message and the Machine

EACH BIOPOLITICAL issue tells us something about who we are and what kind of a world we inhabit. The disputes about species extinction and genetic erosion and biotechnology tell us that the biological nature of the planet is rapidly changing and that the changes are human doing; the new issues of human reproduction tell us that the business of propagating our own kind is not what it used

UNIVERSAL DECLARATION OF THE RIGHTS OF ANIMALS

PREAMBLE
Whereas all animals have rights,
Whereas disregard and contempt for the rights of animals have
resulted and continue to result in crimes by man against nature
and against animals,
Whereas recognition by the human species of the right to existence of
other animal species is the foundation of the co-existence of species
throughout the world,
Whereas genocide has been perpetrated by man on animals and the
threat of genocide continues,
Whereas respect for animals is linked to the respect of man for men,
Whereas from childhood, man should be taught to observe,
understand, respect and love animals,

IT IS HEREBY PROCLAIMED

ARTICLE 1
All animals are born with an equal claim on life and the same rights
to existence.
ARTICLE 2
1) All animals are entitled to respect.
2) Man as an animal species shall not arrogate to himself the right to
exterminate or inhumanely exploit other animals. It is his duty to use
his knowledge for the welfare of animals.
3) All animals have the right to the attention, care and protection of
man.
ARTICLE 3
1) No animal shall be ill-treated or be subject to cruel acts.
2) If an animal has to be killed, this must be instantaneous and
without distress.
ARTICLE 4
1) All wild animals have the right to liberty in their natural
environment, whether land, air or water, and should be allowed
to procreate.
2) Deprivation of freedom, even for educational purposes, is an
infringement of this right.
ARTICLE 5
1) Animals of species living traditionally in a human environment
have the right to live and grow at the rhythm and under the
conditions of life and freedom peculiar to their species.
2) Any interference by man with this rhythm or these conditions
for purposes of gain is an infringement of this right.

[230]

ARTICLE 6

1) All companion animals have the right to complete their natural life span.

2) Abandonment of an animal is a cruel and degrading act.

ARTICLE 7

All working animals are entitled to a reasonable limitation of the duration and intensity of their work, to the necessary nourishment and to rest.

ARTICLE 8

1) Animal experimentation involving physical or psychological suffering is incompatible with the rights of animals, whether it be for scientific, medical, commercial or any other form of research.

2) Replacement methods must be used and developed.

ARTICLE 9

Where animals are used in the food industry they shall be reared, transported, caged and killed without the infliction of suffering.

ARTICLE 10

1) No animal shall be exploited for the amusement of man.

2) Exhibitions and spectacles involving animals are incompatible with their dignity.

ARTICLE 11

Any act involving the wanton killing of an animal is biocide, that is, a crime against life.

ARTICLE 12

1) Any act involving the mass killing of wild animals is genocide, that is, a crime against the species.

2) Pollution or destruction of the natural environment leads to genocide.

ARTICLE 13

1) Dead animals shall be treated with respect.

2) Scenes of violence involving animals shall be banned from cinema and television, except for humane education.

ARTICLE 14

1) Representatives of movements that defend animal rights should have an effective voice at all levels of government.

2) The rights of animals, like human rights, should enjoy the protection of law.

to be; and the animal rights movement tells us about one of several ways in which the social order itself—the moral community, the polis—is changing. This can be looked at either as an expansion of the boundaries to include other living things, or an expansion *within* the boundaries in which human political systems develop new legal protections for living things that once had no status except that of property.

This development overlaps with the concerns of global genetic change, especially species extinction; and converges—to an extent that I would not care to predict—with changing cultural values about nutrition and health. The animal rights cause is helped along greatly by information that (a) meat is not as good for people as was once thought, and (b) that the production of meat is a great consumer of water and energy and agricultural land. The influential book *Diet for a Small Planet*, for example, had nothing to say about animal rights and made its case for vegetarian eating entirely with reference to issues of ecosystem management and human social justice—arguing that meat production squanders resources and is an obstacle to the development of an agriculture that will feed the world's growing population and improve the lot of poorer nations.

Many people are either cutting down on meat-eating or eliminating it entirely for reasons different from those of the animal rights people. This gives the whole subject a certain fluidity, weakens the grip of the meat-eating lifestyle in a way that one movement alone could not. We have, then, non-animal rights vegetarians and animal rights people who continue to eat meat but support reforms in the food factories. We have people who advocate animal rights from a utilitarian position, people who advocate them from a belief in their inherent value, and people who think the whole animal-rights case is overblown but that there should be reforms and protections anyway. Such a complexity of positions might not satisfy the moral purist, but it is politically fertile, a Vavilov center of change and possibility.

It is a mistake to think of animal rights merely as a problem requiring a solution—even though it is indeed a problem and there are indeed solutions, at least partial ones. It is one of the human species' transcendent problems, one that comes with the territory—more precisely, with the econiche; like other dilemmas of evolutionary governance now emerging into our field of vision, it is not about to go away.

I expect the animal rights cause will continue to make progress, but the moral stridency of some activists will also make enemies. Resistance to the cause is formidable and not confined to certain groups like factory farmers and laboratory experimenters. I recently read, in my local newspaper, an op-ed piece by a California political writer, known for his work on environmental issues, who had this to say:

> The indifference that many people of good conscience display toward the cause of animal rights doesn't derive from a lack of sympathy for its objective; it's more a matter of a discomfort with its sense of priorities. Why, after all, at a time when the nuclear shadow is lengthening and the sum of human misery seems to be rising on every hand, are our elected leaders and journals of opinion spending so much time in debating the well-being of rats and mice?[25]

More recently I came across a piece in a newsletter published by the editors of *Mother Jones* which was even more revealing. The article was an explanation of why that magazine, ordinarily an enthusiastic champion of all forms of progressive political activism, had held back on animal rights, refused to cover the subject. It said:

> *Mother Jones* is, remember, a political magazine. The right animal story for us must, therefore, go beyond the rather narrow, knee-jerk antivivisectionist, highly moral positions taken by many animal rights advocates, a number of whom are either committed misanthropes, closet mammalian chauvinists, or guilt-ridden yuppies fatigued with human politics.[26]

Both these statements—the *Mother Jones* one quite explicitly—reflect a view that the animal rights cause, whatever its moral commendability, is not really *politics* at all. Politics is taken to be properly defined as something involving the immediate needs of people. The job of stretching the boundaries of the polis is clearly far from complete. The gun-loving right remains unconverted, and so do members of the environmentalist center and the progressive left as well.

Probably the strongest appeal to the public has to do with animal experimentation for scientific purposes. When we cheer for a malaria vaccine that may save millions of human lives, we are—whether we know it or not—consenting to the use of many thousands of mice and other animals in the research and testing that make such a vaccine possible. At a recent panel on animal rights a scientist pointed out that without the use of laboratory animals we would be without:

[234]

(a) open heart surgery and other major corrective surgery,

(b) organ transplant surgery,

(c) most vaccines and antibiotics,

(d) the prospect of correcting genetic disorders (gene therapy),

(e) virtually all drugs, at the level of safety and efficacy now guaranteed,

(f) the knowledge of carcinogenicity of many pesticides and other chemicals,

(g) birth control pills,

(h) diagnostic tests for infectious diseases involving antibodies,

(i) knowledge of the safety of food additives, cosmetics, many chemicals,

(j) virtually all veterinary medicines and procedures.[27]

Undoubtedly some people are prepared to give up some of the above. But I doubt that most are prepared to give up all of them. Animal experimentation can be reduced and made more humane, and there is much talk of possible alternatives such as cell and organ-culture technology and computer simulation.[28] And yet experimentation goes on, and will continue to go on.

Another difficulty in the way of the animal rights case is that the prospective convert discovers upon closer inspection that there *is* no single point of view to be accepted once one has opened up to the plight of animals. The boundaries remain blurred: What about insects? What about bacteria? I brush my teeth and take countless lives, floss them and destroy habitat. What about plants? Do they suffer? Do they not have inherent value? I read pamphlets proclaiming that no life is to be destroyed, and wonder where the paper came from.

[235]

Such considerations provide an escape for those who would prefer to ignore the whole matter, but actually it is not so arcane as to prevent ordinary people from forming an opinion. We are not sure about the experience of a tree, but the experience of a cat with its spinal cord exposed while scientists drop weights upon it is somewhere within our range of imagination. The subject is accessible to human reason and human compassion, but that does not make it clear and simple; moral questions never are. The essence of moral life in our time is to be deprived of certainty but required to take stands.

Many people take their stand by opting out of arrangements that involve the exploitation of animal life. Vegetarianism—in its various forms—is one way to do this. It has an operational impact by reducing somewhat the profit of the meat industry, and it has a psychological impact for the vegetarian of feeling to have escaped from the burden of sin. "Meatless, Guiltless," proclaimed a *New York Times Magazine* article.[29]

But it isn't that easy. You can be meatless, but guiltlessness is harder to come by. The members of Animal Rights Network, the laboratory-raiding guerrillas of the movement, come closer to guiltlessness by refusing to wear leather shoes or wool clothes, anything made from animals. Yet they are still not apart from the system of interconnections that links the life of every human being to the animals that provide our food and leather, test our medicines and cosmetics and surgical procedures and household products, and in countless ways contribute to our comfort and survival.

None of us in the modern world is separate from this vast system. Our biological existence is connected to that of the animals. They are a part of us, and we of them.

[236]

And it will be difficult indeed to ignore completely the argument that where a biological connection exists, a moral connection exists also.

The future will not be easy for those who embrace the animal rights cause and try to bring its issues within the scope of human politics. It will be hard for those who embrace their cause, it will be hard for those who do not, and it will continue to be hard—who can say how hard, or for how long?—for the millions of living things that are the object of our deliberation.

[7]

Managing a Biosphere:
The Project Begins

ALL OF the challenges and adventures that we have been considering in the foregoing chapters, from navigating the genetic rapids to regulating sperm banks and legislating animal rights, are parts of what I have described as the master challenge of our era. They are being dealt with as many separate political issues, but when taken together—and especially when considered on a global scale—they become not just a new bunch of issues but a force transforming politics itself.

The larger challenge is not the creation of any individual thinker nor the agenda of any single movement. It is not of the same order as other adventures of the human species—such as, say, the exploration of space—that could either be done or left undone indefinitely. Rather it comes upon us in the night as a gathering of necessities. Many people here and there see certain things that must be done, and gradually those discoveries come together into a recognition of a large and unavoidable common cause.

There are many dimensions to the project, but the part that has come the farthest in the direction of being conceptualized is that of maintaining the ecological health of the biosphere. It is not hard to grasp the immediacy of the need to take care of the basic environmental supports of life on Earth, the air and the water and the soil and the forests. This need is so pressing, its urgency growing so rapidly, that it has already thrown the world into an entirely new kind of political crisis. Current threats to the integrity of the biosphere add up to an immense and unprecedented task for governmental institutions, no less urgent than the threat of nuclear warfare. We have grown accustomed to thinking of peacekeeping as the paramount global cause, the herculean chore of political leadership, but Earthkeeping is of equal importance. We could dismantle the war machines tomorrow and discover to our surprise that the world we had saved from nuclear catastrophe was acutely vulnerable to several other forms of destruction from other manifestations of human progress. The imperatives of environmental management goad us toward the creation of a global system of governance— some kind of a managerial arrangement to curtail species extinction and genetic erosion, enable the human population to feed and house itself, permit development, and leave a few options open for future generations.

This sounds like a tall order. It is hard to find even a small region that is a reasonably good example of ecological governance, combining social justice for its human population with good management of its biological resources. Yet the realities of the times demand global ecological— and evolutionary—governance. Such is the human condition: The trains start arriving when we are in the early stages of thinking about how to build a railway station.

The situation, thus stated, sounds rather bleak—and, in many ways, it is. The general level of awareness of the problems and possibilities is not high among the world's political leaders, and the human ability to avoid knowing the truth about its own ecological interventionism is nothing less than stunning. If you have your hopes set on a sudden species-wide change of heart that will bring forth a grand and altruistic global government like the one Tennyson described—"where the war drum throbbed no longer and the battle flags were furled/In the Parliament of Man, the Federation of the world"—you had better be a very patient person, and good at dealing with disappointment. But although signs of such a world government are hard to find, working structures of world governance are rapidly coming into existence. In some respects the new world order is already here; it just doesn't look like one.

We resist seeing the extent of the changes that have taken place in the world political order in the same way—and for some of the same reasons—that we resist seeing the extent of the human interventions that have made such changes necessary. But as the accumulation of information overwhelms our fears, as we acknowledge the true power of human management of the biosphere, we begin to perceive that the thoughts and actions of many people are already harnessed in the service of the project, and that new organizations have come into being for the same larger purpose.

Creeping Globalism

CONSERVATIVES are much given to fretting over "creeping socialism"—the tendency of liberal governments to drift toward collectivist policies that end up looking very much like outright Marxism. The fear is not entirely misplaced, but you can find equally persuasive evidence of a tendency to drift the other way: creeping free-market capitalism. Several Western democracies have shown a tendency to creep left for a few years, then to creep right for a while—locked into an indecisive oscillation between the polarities of Industrial Revolution politics. The pattern is not circular, however; there is a prevailing general direction. The larger drift is not toward global socialism or a global open market, but simply toward a global economy, one in which Marxist national governments open their doors to multinational corporations and governments of all ideological persuasions find it possible to do business with one another even while they remain rhetorically at odds.

There are many globalizing forces at work today: It is generally recognized that we are witnessing the emergence of a new global economy and a global culture as well. It is not, however, quite so generally recognized that there are biological globalizing forces at work, and that we are also witnessing the emergence of a new kind of global ecosystem.

The world has always been a biological unit in a certain sense, and many writers who have puzzled over its mysterious existence have come to the conclusion that it is something very like an organism. But like all organisms it has many parts that seem to have lives of their own, and the natural sciences have paid a great deal of attention to the kinds of parts we call ecosystems—communities of plant and animal life, occupying a certain geographical space. An ecosystem, like a nation, has boundaries, but—and here is where natural scientists show a good deal more common sense than statesmen—it is understood that such boundaries are shifting, loose, and permeable. An ecosystem is linked to other ecosystems, contained within larger systems in the rich and infinitely complex structure of life. A pond ecosystem is part of the deep geological structure of the land it occupies, and also part of the region's river system and weather system and—if migrating birds spend some time there—of that larger pattern as well. The organizational structure of nature is multidimensional and multifaceted: wheels within wheels, systems overlapping and interacting, systems of different sizes and different kinds, all of them changing in both cyclical and linear transitions.

The natural events of life continually alter ecosystems. A new species appears in an area and bumps another out of its econiche; a predator dies off from a disease while the animals it preys on undergo a population explosion and decimate their favorite plants; a migrating bird drops a seed that grows into an aggressively spreading plant. The appearance of human life is at first only the entry of another actor onto the scene—but then the rambling bipeds begin to increase both the geographic reach and the rate of speed of ecological change—and also do so for entirely new reasons. Immigrants to the New World brought plants and animals for agriculture—and they also brought fish and wildlife for sport, and other plants and animals just for the hell of it. American history is rich with stories of people who contributed to the remodeling of its ecosystems on the basis of little more than whim.

Whatever mode of transportation happens to be, at any given time, the state-of-the-art means of human movement becomes also the medium for establishing new transplants: When people had no means of movement but their feet, they strolled from place to place with seeds and cuttings and domesticated animals; when they had sailing ships, they carried plants and animals about the world; now we have jets, and they connect ecosystems as well as airports.

The new ecological reality of the world is being simultaneously discovered and created. We are finding out that past human actions caused ecological transformations that extend over a far greater reach of time and space than we had previously believed, and that these transformations have produced new political problems and forged connections between people—and plants and animals and insects—who once had very little to do with one another; at the same time further actions with even greater impacts are being set in motion, producing new problems and new linkages.

Modern transportation and communications and commerce, human migrations, and the biological manipulations of agriculture and science are wrapping a new system of linkages around the globe, creating new patterns of interaction among all the things that inhabit it. The effects of human civilization sweep through all natural ecosystems, change them, and connect them in new ways to the rest of the world. This was what I meant by saying (in Chapter One) that the various advances of human civilization—such as the discovery of evolution itself—are whole-system transitions. They alter not only the way people think, but the biological conditions of the entire planet.

The genetic rapids is the result of multiple alterations of the biosphere. The human forces behind these vary from accidents—chiefly secondary results of population growth—to the deliberate and complex manipulations of modern biotechnology. Whatever the cause, the effect is modification of the total gene pool—changes in the genetic information available to be communicated to future generations of life on Earth.

Another category of changes are alterations of land ecosystems: deforestation, soil erosion, changes in water systems, floods. In the Himalayas, growing populations range farther and farther in search of firewood, destroying watersheds, and the resultant floods rage down hundreds of miles to Bangladesh. In Central America, tropical rains wash away the topsoil from worn-out hillside farms, silt up hydroelectric projects that embody national hopes to produce cheap power, and flood fertile lowland regions.

Central America, wasted by centuries of colonial agriculture and careless land use, shows vividly the pattern that is repeated with variations through much of the Third World. El Salvador, the most ravaged and crowded country in the region—90 percent deforested, a population density higher than India's—has been importing firewood and exporting hungry and unemployed people for decades. The refugee problem led to a war with neighboring Honduras in the 1960s, when the refugees were expelled. Today Salvadorean refugees are in Honduras again, and in other Central American countries, and in Mexico and the United States. When a country's life support systems become as seriously damaged as those of El Salvador, there are inevitable impacts on neighboring countries: an outflow of people, an inflow of basic goods such as firewood. These impacts become more serious when the neighboring countries are also experiencing rapid population growth, deforestation, and soil erosion; the result is something like the famous "domino theory" of the Vietnam war days, except that here the consequences are spreading ecological collapse, with economic hardships, political unrest and more landless migrants heading toward the sprawling urban slums and the borders of El Norte. This process is not, strictly speaking, global—except that it is happening in many places around the world, and that wherever it occurs it has regional and international consequences.

The most clearly global changes are those affecting the parts of the world organism that transcend national boundaries and connect to all terrestial life. We hear of increasing carbon dioxide in the atmosphere and of likely increases in the Earth's temperature from the greenhouse effect. We hear of nitrogen compounds (from agricultural fertilizers, aerosol spray vapors, and the emissions of jet airplanes) in the stratosphere, where they destroy the ozone layer which controls the amount of ultraviolet radiation let into the atmosphere. Ultraviolet radiation is absorbed by DNA and protein molecules, and a major fluctuation would undoubtedly have biological effects. Nobody knows precisely what they might be, or what levels of nitrogen compounds might produce a major change in the conditions of life on the planet's surface. We hear of worldwide acid pollution—not just acid rain, but acidification spreading in mist and dry air, in melting snow, and through the soil itself. Again, we cannot precisely identify the causes or predict the consequences—although it is clear that a wide range of human activities contribute to it, and a wide range of ecological and economic problems are likely to be its results.[1]

The causes and effects of biochemical change in the oceans are better understood, and constitute our most serious threat to a part of the global ecological infrastructure. No matter how far nations proclaim their boundaries to extend outward from their shorelines, the ocean remains a common resource of all life—and one that is clearly not in the best of health. It has always served as humanity's garbage can at the same time that it has served as a major source of food—two functions whose incompatability is becoming ever more apparent. Today we are asking the sea to absorb uncomplainingly into its vast depths a colossal amount of wastes: sewage of huge cities, toxic outpourings of factories, water from polluted rivers, oil from tankers, containers of atomic garbage. Meanwhile the fishing vessels range over the waters, decimating the fisheries in search of food to meet the ever-growing human demand and bringing some species of marine life to the brink of extinction.

These are, strictly speaking, biological events and not political ones. They become political events when information about them accumulates and becomes public knowledge. It is this information-generating process I want to look at in this chapter, rather than the underlying ecological problems that the information is about, because information gives rise to global organization. Feedback—in this case data about a human society's effects on its environment—is the essence of evolutionary governance.

The First Global Report

THE NEED for political systems to manage the global commons in the public interest (a public now expanding to include future generations and non-human entities, the whole community of life) grows in direct relationship to human capacity to intervene in nature and alter ecosystems. The need did not exist at all when human numbers were small and technology primitive; it emerged gradually with the development of civilization.

In fact there *was* no global commons until there were systems of human interaction that connected different parts of the world, and information technology that gave people an idea of a biosphere and some knowledge about what they were doing to it. As human numbers increase, as we intervene more, and as we become more capable of knowing the consequences of our interventions, we begin to see the ways people and ecosystems are being linked together—and perceive that a global commons exists. Knowledge of large-scale impacts will tend to bring global governance into being whether we want it or not. Information creates global environmentalism.

The present-day Information Revolution is not the first tidal wave of knowledge and power that has transformed ecosystems and governments. The discovery of America—which was really the discovery of the globe—was itself a great consciousness-raiser, and a necessary prelude to the era of colonialism, which in turn produced a period of rapid increase in the transplantation of life forms, human and non-human. (I was fascinated to discover some years ago that the original use of the word "plantation" was to denote a plantation of human settlers in a new location.)

But while human impacts upon the Earth increased both in kind and in global reach, few people comprehended that they were in fact re-making the world. There was no ecological science as such, no concept of secondary and tertiary effects. The extent of the changes taking place were not comprehended, and people seem to have generally assumed that domesticated regions were more stable.

These attitudes underwent steady erosion—the word serves well here—throughout the nineteenth century. Disturbing news came in from many directions. Some scientists reported on large-scale ecological changes that were taking place in distant parts of the British empire as a result of the land-use patterns—deforestation and the creation of huge plantations (of coffee and cotton and tobacco and tea, as well as people)—that served colonial trade. Some discovered new historical evidence that there had been striking transformations of the Mediterranean region caused by the ancient Greeks and Romans. Particularly disturbing news came from the Alps, a region Europeans thought of as their great wilderness.

Beginning late in the eighteenth century and increasing through the following decades, European geographers published several studies indicating that the destructive Alpine torrents that flooded the farms and settlements of the lowlands were the result of deforestation in the mountains. Some investigators claimed that the logging was not only altering the river systems and ruining agricultural areas far from the high forests, but was changing the climate of the entire region. The people who read such reports—many scientists, a few public officials—began to struggle with unfamiliar ideas: ecosystems that were not respecters of political boundaries, long-range effects over time and space, huge and half-accidental modifications of the Earth's surface.

The news arrived in bits and pieces, in many separate studies, and few people put the pieces together. Charles Darwin did not. Neither did his mentor in the earth sciences, the English geologist Charles Lyell. The person who did put the pieces together—and who deserves to be remembered as an equal to Darwin in the human species' great adventure in discovering the truth about itself—was an American, George Perkins Marsh. In his monumental work *Man and Nature, or, Physical Geography as Modified by Human Action*, first published in 1864, Marsh summarized the results of a huge amount of research (he read 20 languages) and painted a vivid picture of a world that was continually changing. The causes of change he identified were ordinary human activities—farming, logging, fire, conversion of land to agriculture, modification of waterways, domestication and movement of plants and animals.[2] His was the first general work to synthesize the findings of specialists such as meteorologists, agronomists, hydrologists, and botanists; he gathered such information together into a picture of what was happening in the world, and gave the picture to the public. Marsh was not a back-to-nature man; he regarded human intervention as necessary and inevitable. But he spoke forcefully for a more prudent management of the Earth's living resources. His book had a great impact in both Europe and the United States. He was, more than anyone else, the source and inspiration of the early conservationist movement, forerunner of modern environmentalism, that reached its peak in the Theodore Roosevelt years. But on the whole, despite the profound impact of Marsh's message, his work was for some time overshadowed by that of Spencer, who wrote of human intervention as a process mainly confined to the cultivated and domesticated portions of the world, rather than a force that was massive, global, and only partially under control. The full impact of Marsh's work was not felt until the present century, when it was supplemented by other ideas that had to do not only with human action but with Earth itself.

Humanity Discovers the Biosphere

IN THE EARLY part of this century a new concept was developed—an idea of Earth as a unified living system, and of human life as something that emerges within that system and transforms it. Such a concept is a necessary prerequisite to the project of global governance that is now emerging. Mainstream Western science and philosophy had lacked any such concept; its origins are connected with the appearance of the word *biosphere*.

That term was coined, rather offhandedly, by an Austrian geologist named Edward Suess in a book about the origin of the Alps.[3] Its development into a way of conceptualizing life on Earth is associated with the Russian mineralogist V.I. Vernadsky, who lectured on the subject and wrote a book entitled *The Biosphere*, published in France in 1929. Vernadsky described the biosphere as a specific portion of the planet, the portion within which life develops; it includes the troposphere (the lower atmosphere), the hydrosphere (the oceans), and the lithosphere (a layer of earth approximately three kilometers deep). This, he said, was the "terrestrial envelope within which life can exist." He described all living matter as genetically connected by having evolved within this envelope; and saw the human species as an organic product of the biosphere, understandable only as a part of its "material and energetic structure."[4]

Vernadsky was influenced by the work of his colleague Alexy Pavlov, who saw the human species as an active geologic force, transforming the biosphere by deliberate and accidental interventions, and indeed by its very presence. Vernadsky was particularly intrigued by the observation that human activity was producing artificial minerals. This view of the human species as an agent in the evolution of the biosphere became a part of Vernadsky's thinking; he later described the process with the word *noosphere*, which had been developed in collaborative work between the French mathematician/philosopher Edouard LeRoy and the theologian/paleontologist Pierre Teilhard de Chardin. That word came into general use after the publication in France in 1938 of Teilhard's *The Phenomenon of Man*. Although Teilhard did not clearly define it, it is generally taken to mean a sphere of mind, something developing within the biosphere and also transforming it and in a sense superseding it—becoming the agent of further stages of evolutionary development.[5]

Vernadsky had no doubt that the appearance of human intelligence in the biosphere was a major evolutionary event whose meaning was just beginning to be comprehended. In an article published just after his death in 1945 he wrote:

> The noosphere is a new geological phenomenon on our planet. In it for the first time man becomes a *large-scale geological force*. He can and must rebuild the province of his life by his work and thought, rebuild it radically in comparison with the past. Wider and wider creative possibilities open before him. It may be that the generation of our grandchildren will approach their blossoming.[6]

The concept did not gain converts quickly. Vernadsky's work was little known outside of the scientific world; Teilhard's *Phenomenon of Man* was a little too religious for many scientists and a little too scientific (and evolutionary) for his superiors in the Church; it was, perhaps most seriously, lacking in concrete specifics about what the human phenomenon was doing or had done or might do in the biosphere. Nevertheless, the pieces of a fundamentally different world-view were in place: the concept of the planet as a unified living system, and the concept of human civilization as a powerful new force within that system, capable of transforming it in any of several directions, and also, quite conceivably, of destroying it. Over the next few decades, those concepts were gradually given new coherence and detail, fleshed out by information, turned into ideas accessible to the public and political leaders, made ready to serve as a new vision of human civilization.

In 1956 a group of scholars came together in Princeton for a symposium on "Man's Role in Changing the Face of the Earth." This conference, convened in Marsh's memory, produced a two-volume study, the most comprehensive work of its sort since Marsh's own pioneering effort—in fact the twentieth century's first complete survey of the record of human intervention and the current condition of the biosphere.[7] The study, and the cadre of world-class environmental scientists and generalists who had produced it (the contributors included Lewis Mumford, Kenneth Boulding, and Teilhard de Chardin) became basic resources of the environmental movement.

In the years immediately following, two worldwide programs of scientific study made further contributions to this growing body of information: These were the International Geophysical Year (1957-58) and the International Biological Programme (1964-74), the latter formed for the specific purpose of taking stock of "the biological basis of productivity and human welfare" on a global scale.

Another step in the discovery of the biosphere—more specifically, a step in the direction of its being discovered by political leaders—was the UNESCO Biosphere Conference. The full title of this conference is worth noting in all its ponderousness, because it gives a sense of the shifting of conceptual gears that was taking place: The 1966 resolution called for an "Intergovernmental Conference of Experts on the Scientific Basis for Rational Use and Conservation of the Resources of the Biosphere." It thus expressed a conventional view of the subject—the "conservation of resources" idea, which was familiar, based in economics, and respectable, even if not widely practiced—and the newer biosphere idea which was based in evolution and ecology.[8] Anybody who goes in for drawing lines between old paradigms and new ones should keep in mind Scott Fitzgerald's famous pronouncement that the test of a first-rate intelligence is the ability to retain two diametrically opposed concepts in the mind at the same time and still retain the ability to function. The conference, held in Paris in September of 1968, produced an action-oriented report, the most forthright document on the world environment *as a single entity and as a matter of urgent political concern* that had ever been adopted by a governmental body. It insisted that old patterns of exploitation "must give way to recognition that the biosphere is a system all of which is widely affected by action on any part of it," and concluded:

Until this point in history the nations of the world have lacked considered comprehensive policies for managing the environment . . . . Although changes have been taking place for a long time, they seem to have reached a threshold recently that has made the public aware of them. This awareness is leading to concern, and to the recognition that to a large degree, man now has the capability and responsibility to determine and

[253]

guide the future of his environment, and to the beginnings of national and international corrective action . . . .[9]

The conservationism of the Theodore Roosevelt era had been, despite the influence of Marsh's global vision, domestic in focus, chiefly concerned about the forests and other natural resources of the American terrain; but the new environmentalism that made its debut around Earth Day of 1971 was unabashedly global. "Earth" was its symbolic seal, the word that expressed both its intellectual and emotional content; it was, almost from the moment of its birth, one of history's few genuinely global political movements.

This globalism flexed its muscles at the 1972 Stockholm conference, convened by the UN General Assembly at about the same time that the Biosphere conference was getting underway in Paris. The Stockholm conference was the first international conference on the environment; this signaled a move of the UN into environmentalism, and it brought together representatives from developed countries and developing countries. The former tended to be concerned about protecting the environment; the latter tended to be concerned about equitable human distribution of its wealth, and were not too sure they wanted to hear about the North's new fad. It was thus the beginning of serious environmental diplomacy. It was also the occasion for an unofficial convention for NGOs: non-governmental organizations concerned with environmental issues. These organizations were really just beginning to emerge as a force in world politics, and they had their own conference while the diplomats were having theirs. The city teemed with scientists, political activists, famous environmentalists, and guitar-toting young devotees of the new movement.

The conference was productive, despite the circus-like atmosphere and the deep cleavage between North and South. One of its products was something that happened even before it convened: Eighty-five nations prepared national reports, most of them the first surveys that the countries had ever made of their environmental conditions and concerns. The conference produced agreement among all of its 113 participant nations on a sizeable list of specific proposals for action. It established the World Environment Fund and created the UN Environmental Programme, headquartered in Nairobi—the first global intergovernmental body with its center located somewhere outside of North America or Europe. Maurice Strong, the conference's secretary-general, said later that, as its outcome, "For the first time we began to see that all mankind literally is in the same boat—that the world community is faced with its first truly global problem."[10] Political scientist Lynton K. Caldwell, appraising the conference ten years after, said that its primary accomplishment was "the identification and legitimization of the biosphere as an object of national and international policy."[11]

Although the word "biosphere" has indeed come into general use, the meaning of the word in all its subversive richness has not yet penetrated into the consciousness of the world leaders who now employ it. It is not easy, after a lifetime of carrying in one's mind a mapmaker's picture of a planet marked off into distinct nation-states, to see it as a single living entity.

If the mapmaker's picture is obsolete, so is the back-to-nature image of a world separated into ecosystems and bioregions. The same human activities that transcend national boundaries also transform and link ecosystems in new ways. Some ecologists, recognizing this, now employ

[255]

the concept of a "noosystem," a holistic approach which includes "not only a study of the structure and function of ecological systems, but also the social, economic and cultural influences on such systems."[12]

Thinking about such things has changed greatly, and will change even more. It is impossible to maintain a conceptual status quo in the midst of an information deluge. The world news keeps coming in.

The Feedback Business

REPORTS ON the status of the biosphere, virtually non-existent until the middle of this century, now issue forth regularly from both governmental and non-governmental sources, continuing to demonstrate the commonality of global environmental concerns. Environmentalism is an information-age phenomenon, a political force whose strength lies more in its data base than in its manifestos.

One of the first of the current crop of global reports was *The Limits to Growth*, the Club of Rome's famous compendium of projections on world population growth, resource use, and food production—information coupled with an urgent message that the path of development then being pursued by most of the world's economic and political leadership was leading straight toward a tangle of shortages and ecological catastrophes.[13]

Limits was published in 1972, the year of the Stockholm Conference; later in the same decade, during the Carter administration, the President's Council on Environmental Quality produced the *Global 2000* report, the U. S. government's first systematic effort to take stock of the state of the biosphere. That report, while less outspoken than *Limits to Growth*, was nevertheless forthright in predicting ecological hard times. "If present trends continue," it warned, "the world in 2000 will be more crowded, more polluted, less stable ecologically, and more vulnerable to disruption than the world we live in now. Serious stresses involving population, resources, and environment are clearly visible ahead." Among the specific forecasts were a variety of obstacles to eliminating poverty in the Third World, regional water shortages in some areas, significant losses of world forests, deterioration of agricultural soils, atmospheric concentrations of carbon dioxide and ozone-depleting chemicals, and extinctions of plant and animal species rising dramatically. "The needed changes," it concluded, "go far beyond the capability and responsibility of this or any other single nation. An era of unprecedented cooperation and commitment is essential."[14]

The *Global 2000* report got a hot-potato treatment by some agencies within the Carter administration that produced it and was condemned to total obscurity by the Reagan administration that followed. Yet it has attained a certain celebrity status among government publications. In conservative circles, it is viewed with great distaste. On the other side, it has become the centerpiece of a network of environmental groups—the Global Tomorrow Coalition—whose purpose is to keep the report's message before the public. In view of the number of publications the U. S. government produces and the complete and well-deserved obscurity most of them attain, it is worth considering why only one publication of recent years has attained such status. What is so special about its content? The answer is not merely that the report criticizes and challenges some of the assumptions about human progress that have prevailed since before the beginning of the Industrial Revolution; that critique is a mild one. The report's real subversiveness lies in its very subject matter, which is the consequences of human intervention, and in its scope: It talks about the biosphere, and every piece of information it advances—be the news good or bad—helps create the global commons.

So the U.S. government's first effort at comprehensive data-gathering became a political liability, and the federal government did not go seriously into the global feedback business. But private organizations did. Notable among them on the Washingon think-tank scene are the Worldwatch Institute, which produces reports on various aspects of the biosphere and an annual book entitled *State of the World*; and the World Resources Institute, which in 1986 published its own global report, *World Resources*. Another is the International Institute for Environment and Development, which is supported by various national governments and international agencies including the United Nations Environmental Programme and the World Bank; IIED's activities include a global news and information service called Earthscan. In 1985 the Global Tomorrow Coalition sponsored the first in a series of "Globescope" conferences to pool and disseminate such information.

Worldwatch, World Resources, Earthscan, Globescope; the names say it all, announce that, whatever political and economic course the human species chooses to follow in the decades to come, it will be harder and harder to pretend ignorance of the consequences.

There is another side to the feedback business. In some circles the literature I have cited above is regarded as alarmist and anti-progress, and a counter-movement aimed at challenging such dour forecasts is in the field. The last book publication from the late futurist Herbert Kahn was an anthology, co-edited with Julian Simon and entitled

The Resourceful Earth: A Response to Global 2000. The various contributions in the book, which could as well have been entitled *Not to Worry*, were arguments that the *Global 2000* report had vastly overstated its case.[15]

Such an effort is a healthy addition to what is now a global dialogue. The quality of information produced by the feedback network is likely to be improved by being challenged, and it is far better that the information be challenged than repressed, as has happened so often with subversive knowledge. The more there is argument about the condition of the global commons, the more the *idea* of a global commons will make itself comfortable squarely in the center of the politics of the decades to come. The presence of such a dialogue—the first real debate about the future of the biosphere—is one of the most important points of interest in the political landscape of our time. Sometimes it is more instructive to take note of what people are arguing about than to try to figure out who is winning the argument.

The organizations and publications I have named here are only a small part of the huge information-gathering and -disseminating apparatus that has come into being around the world in the past few decades. There are other private organizations and scientific groups, as well as spec-ialized books and magazines, television documentaries, and newspaper articles. There are international assessment programs, such as the UN's Global Environmental Mon-itoring System (GEMS) and International Referral System (INFOTERRA), the latter a kind of dating service that gets people who need information in touch with people who have it. As I write, yet another program is getting underway. Preliminary plans are now in the works for an International Geosphere-Biosphere Program (IGBP) which will be a step beyond all the other global studies—will be, in fact, the largest coordinated scientific project ever undertaken. It will study the Earth's core, the condition of ecosystems on land and sea, and the global climate. It will provide the best available information about global threats such as ozone depletion and the greenhouse effect. The organizing committee hopes that it will also produce a new discipline—"Earth system science"—based on the study of how such processes interact.

Other information-gathering initiatives are underway in relation to genetic resources and endangered species. Several other countries are developing computerized national genetic resource inventories comparable to the U.S. network, and already there is talk—paralleling the move in the FAO for free exchange of genetic material—about a global system for free exchange of information on what resources exist in gene banks and where they are located. Scientists have been naming and cataloging species for centuries, but we still lack a clear idea of the diversity of life on Earth. Edward Wilson (among others) now proposes "nothing less than a full count, a complete catalog of life on Earth." Wilson says that a complete survey, while admittedly a huge task of research and information processing, is well within the range of possibility: "Compared with what has been dared and achieved in high-energy physics, molecular genetics, and other branches of 'big science,' it is in the second or third rank."[16]

If we put all the pieces together, we see a huge database coming into being. It will be not only *about* the global commons but will also be a part of it, a public resource and an element in global governance. The state, we observed earlier, is an information system; as a global information system develops it creates a *de facto* governance system.

The Organization Explosion

ALONG WITH the other sequences of events that can be described by an exponential curve, we must include the increase in the number of organizations in the world. Today there are a lot more of them—organizations of all kinds, but most importantly, organizations that are international or multinational in scope, that have global interests and are players on the world stage. In the decades since the end of World War II, a new system of global interaction has come into being, almost unnoticed. Only a part of this system has arisen out of deliberate attempts by political leaders to create a framework for global cooperation; the growth of global governance is a much more diverse and complex phenomenon, and it is a system with so many odd parts and new players that we may be disinclined to view it as a system at all.

Let us begin by considering the basic component of this global system, the nation-state. The modern nation-state is, however contradictory this might sound, essentially an organization created for international purposes. A society that is not interested in what is going on elsewhere around the world and not worried about its neighbors does not need a national government; it can make do with much simpler arrangements. The nation-state arises in order to perform such tasks as defending its territory from invasion, protecting and promoting the commercial aspirations of its citizens, and giving its political elites international status. Nationalism in the United States has always been bound up with such international aspirations as Manifest Destiny, the Monroe Doctrine, and international commerce, even when the country considered itself isolationist.

Since the end of World War II, the number of recognized "sovereign" nation-states in the world has grown from about 50 to over 200. These are, with few standoffish exceptions, active international participants, with embassies around the world, trade and tourism relations with other countries, and representatives at the United Nations.

The rise of international organizations is equally striking. Over the same period of time, the number of intergovernmental organizations (IGOs) has grown from about 80 to about 400. Most nation-states are great joiners and belong to many of these—regional associations, defense alliances, economic associations. Among them are such major world actors as the North Atlantic Treaty Organization, the Organization for Economic Co-operation and Development, and the Organization of Petroleum Exporting Countries. Regional bodies include the Organization of American States, the Organization of African Unity, and the Association of Southeast Asian Nations. There is the British Commonwealth, the European Economic Community, the Arab League, and the Warsaw Pact. There is the United Nations and its various specialized and related agencies, such as the International Labor Organization, the Food and Agriculture Organization, the World Health Organization, and the International Monetary Fund. Such bodies, floating out there in the distant alphabet soup of international politics, may seem to many of us to be little more than meaningless bureaucracies, and it is true that some of them are—but the permanent international organization is an important part of modern world governance, a sign that the world has changed greatly from the time when nations interacted with one another only through the exchange of ambassadors, bilateral *ad hoc* negotiations, and the occasional treaty conference.

A third major category of actors on the global scene is multinational business. Global trade is not new, but the multinational or transnational corporations—with their subsidiaries all over the world, and their ability to move funds from country to country, to locate plants wherever labor prices are low and the legal climate favorable—are both new and different. They are, in a way, stateless organizations, but they are also engaged in governance: management of the biosphere and interventions in evolution. They are making decisions about land use; operating farms; selling seeds; manufacturing agricultural chemicals and machinery; creating and marketing biotechnology products; breeding animals; processing food and fiber; creating new methods of plant, animal and human reproduction; and financing research and development in every field. The multinationals are viewed as more or less equivalent to the forces of evil by many people on the left, and on the other side I occasionally meet people who believe that the upper levels of multinational management represent the only place where true vision and world leadership can be found, and that if anybody is capable of steering the evolution of the planet it is those brilliant men and women in the board rooms. I am not exaggerating, by the way; no class of organization inspires such feelings in both directions. The multinationals are among the more interesting parts of the new global system, if for no other reason than that they have made it clear that one era in human political evolution is ended: The nation-states are no longer the only organizations with clout in global politics, and may not even be the most important.

[263]

The fourth category in this new system is comprised of NGOs, non-governmental organizations. In *GAIA: An Atlas of Planet Management*, there is a graphic depiction of their rise; it is, sure enough, an exponential curve, moving steeply upward from 1910 when a couple hundred groups qualified as international NGOs (active in three or more countries), to 1983 when there were close to 5000. The authors note that with the addition of organizations of related categories (such as religious bodies and nongovernmental organizations based in a single country but with an international orientation) the number rises to over 12,000.[17] Nowhere in the system is the primacy of biospherical concerns more apparent than here. Such groups as the International Union for the Conservation of Nature, the International Planned Parenthood Fund, and the World Wildlife Fund are among those with a clear and explicit mission to influence public policy toward the biosphere; others such as Oxfam, with its orientation toward food and agriculture, and the International Council of Scientific Unions, which oversaw the International Biological Programme, are also integral parts of the governance system.

It would be nice to be able to report that this amazing tangle of new organizations is at work preserving the biosphere. It isn't, of course. Some parts of it are, but many of the organizations are at work destroying the biosphere, and the great majority of them came into being with no conscious evolutionary or ecological agendas. We need to keep in mind that the whole global/environmental connection in world politics is very, very recent. While the organizational explosion has been going on for approximately forty years, the concept of the biosphere has been in use among world political leaders only during the last twenty, since environmentalism suddenly emerged as a global political movement. Yet the whole international system has become increasingly occupied with biosphere management, and many parts of it exist exclusively for such purposes.

I have spoken of this odd, multidimensional melange of nations and IGOs and NGOs and corporations as a system, and it is that aspect of it that most needs to be understood. It is not news that government and business, for all the mythos of the separation of the public sector from the private sector, are quite interdependent. John Kenneth Gailbraith put it nicely in *The New Industrial State* when he said that "the line between public and private authority in the industrial system is indistinct and in large measure imaginary, and the abhorrent association of public and private organizations is normal."[18] This truth abut the industrial state is equally applicable to the information-era and biopolitical global polis, expanded to include IGOs and NGOs. The system is knitting itself together so rapidly, in fact, that it has produced serious moves toward reversing or at least slowing the process.

The Retreat from Globalism

CREEPING globalism has not yet reached the point of being as fervently opposed as creeping socialism, but the rollback effort is definitely underway. It is a political force somewhat similar to the old American isolationism that arose with such power after World War I and scuttled Woodrow Wilson's dreams for the League of Nations—but this time it is facing a stronger globalizing trend, and is likely to grow into a more formidable counter-trend.

Rollback is a process that people who are hoping for a quick transformation of society seldom take seriously. They reduce history to trends and megatrends, and pay little attention to the rule that any movement of any import invariably produces a counter-movement, and that often those counter-movements prove to be remarkably effective. Note, for example, the accomplishments of Prince Clemens Metternich, the nineteenth-century architect of rollback, whose political career was dedicated, with considerable success, to stemming the tide of republican revolution and restoring Europe to the status quo of rule by monarchy. Or consider the work of latter-day counterforce tacticians such as John Foster Dulles and Henry Kissinger (the latter an avowed admirer of Metternich) who did so much to shape the anti-Communist thrust that is still the chief (and sometimes the only) visible overall direction of U.S. foreign policy. The tenacity of such movements should give pause to anyone who believes that the power structures of the world are about to be effortlessly swept away on a fresh breeze of global environmentalism.

For every globalizing force at work in the world today, there is a corresponding counterforce—not necessarily an equal one, but in every case one worthy of respect. Economic globalization is opposed by industrial policies and protectionism, and by appeals to economic nationalism of the "buy American" variety. Cultural globalization is opposed by retreats into cultural traditionalism and religious fundamentalism. Global migration is countered by moves to control immigration. Global movement of plants and animals is countered by national policies and by international agreements such as the Convention on International Trade in Endangered Species.

To further complicate the matter, we have counter-movements within counter-movements. Nationalism is the greatest single ideological force against globalism, but nationalism itself was a revolutionary movement in its own time, seeking to unite diverse ethnic and religious groups—and it is far from having won its own battle. There are few modern nation-states of any size that do not have to contend with separatist movements of peoples aspiring to go their own way as Basques, Palestinians, Welshmen, French Canadians, etc. Another counter-movement is the "bioregionalism" among some environmentalists, who hope for the salvation of the biosphere through a devolution to simpler and smaller units where people know the characteristics of their local ecosystems and live in harmony with them.

All these can be expected to be a part of the political picture in the decades ahead, but the most serious conflict, the real struggle for the biosphere, will be the kind that emerged around the Law of the Sea Treaty. This showed the United States at its schizoid best, very much like the country that made its entry onto the world stage at the end of World War I by first browbeating its allies into the creation of the League of Nations and then declining to join same. It also showed the real polarization—far more important than the familiar capitalist-communist one—in the new global politics of biosphere management: the polarization between North and South, developed nations vs. developing nations, rich vs. poor. In this polarization, the U.S. has taken the leadership against internationalist moves—such as the UN Industrial Development Organization's international biotechnology center and the Food and Agriculture Organization's convention on exchange of genetic information—that would establish organizations parallel to those controlled by multinational business.

The internationally-controlled deep-sea mining consortium called Enterprise, which was part of the Law of the Sea Treaty, was conceptually very much like the above. Under the treaty, the International Seabed Authority would have been required to permit seabed mineral development both by private mining companies (or the state companies of socialist nations) and also by the international consortium, which, it was understood, would be operated by and for the developing nations.

I do not mean to indicate, to those readers who may not be familiar with the details of this rather sad chapter in the history of evolutionary governance, that the Law of the Sea treaty only had to do with deep-sea mining. That is the rock upon which it crashed and the aspect of it that got the most attention in the media, but mining was only a small part of the package. The treaty was the product of a monumental diplomatic effort, an international conference that had gone on for the better part of a decade, with delegates from over 150 nations hammering out agreement upon a host of problems concerning that great centerpiece of the global commons, the world's oceans.

Although the Law of the Sea Conference (actually the event we are talking about was the third such conference) never had anything like the glitter and publicity surrounding the great conference at Versailles that produced the League of Nations, or the celebrated gathering at San Francisco where the United Nations was born, it was by every other measure the equal of them both: In many ways, it was humanity's greatest effort at constitutionalizing international governance.

The Third Law of the Sea Conference began with an astounding agenda: ocean pollution, navigation through crowded international straits, scientific research, conservation of fisheries, protection of marine mammals, offshore oil drilling, and global standardization of territorial claims. The main goals were (a) to consolidate the vast body of laws and treaties and practices and agreements that had grown up over the centuries in regard to the sea, (b) to address newer concerns such as increasing ocean traffic, pollution, and depletion of some fisheries, and (c) to bring some order out of the chaos of claims of different nations as to how far their territorial waters extended. The conferees reached agreement on all points, and there was every reason to expect that the resultant treaty would be signed and ratified by the United States. The conference had been launched with enthusiastic U.S. support, and had proceeded under three presidents (Nixon, Ford, and Carter); the U.S. delegation had been mainly under Republican leadership. There had been some grumbling from U.S. mining companies about the seabed minerals proposals, but the "two track" idea had come from the U.S.—was part of a package called the "Kissinger compromises," in fact—and the mining companies stood to do well under the agreement. But the negotiations continued into the administration of a fourth president, Ronald Reagan, who decided not to sign the Convention.

"I kind of thought," President Reagan said upon announcing his decision to back out on the product of years of diplomacy, "that when you go out on the high seas, you can do what you want."[19] An Australian diplomat told a reporter: "A wave of dismay has gone around the world."[20]

Dissatisfaction with the seabed mining arrangement was the surface reason for the rejection, but underlying that was a more generalized ideological distrust of global agencies responsive to Third World interests. There had been some talk rumbling about the world concerning the need for a "New International Economic Order" (NIEO) to improve the lot of developing nations, and the Reagan administration chose to see the Law of the Sea treaty as a domino that would send the future toppling in that direction. A White House policy paper said that the treaty would:

> ... transfer control of the ocean's minerals to an international authority dominated by Third World states, which are largely hostile to free market approaches and to the interests of the industrialized nations of the free world .... The LOS treaty is viewed by the (developing countries) as a significant step toward ... the establishment of a NIEO, ... a scheme for restructuring the international eonomy along the socialist lines of the world's centrally managed economies and for redistributing the world's wealth.[21]

Thus, as seen from Washington, socialism and globalism creep together.

The Law of the Sea episode is richly illustrative of what happens as the human species moves seriously and consciously into global governance. It contains both the good news and the bad: It shows that the majority of the world's governments recognize the need for new arrangements to integrate the system and are prepared to invest hugely of time and effort and money in efforts to create them. It shows that even in highly complex sets of issues people can create arrangements to reconcile the aspirations of nation-states and multinational corporations and nongovernmental organizations—can combine solutions to ancient political problems such as territorial waters with ecosystem management, pollution control, and endangered species protection. That is the good news. The bad news is that such efforts can be opposed and derailed, much as was the world's first effort at building a permanent international peacekeeping body.

Toward an Ecology of Governance

WHAT WE are seeing, in this rather confusing back-and-forth shuffle of political developments, is the emergence of a global system of governance. This is the new polis, a system brought into being incrementally—one piece here, another there—to deal with the common responsibilities we share in this envelope of life that Vernadsky described, to define and carry out our intentions toward the troposphere and the hydrosphere and the lithosphere. We have never created a global system of governance before, and obviously a lot of people, Tennyson included, thought it would look a lot different. But this is it. The project has begun.

The central point of the concept of the biosphere is that life on Earth is a single system. The central point of the concept of the noosphere is that human civilization is also a system. Its parts link, interact, and develop in response to one another. This process accelerates with improvements in information flow and transportation; we are really just seeing the system come into being—and discovering that it is a system—in the present era. The human species has, in a burst of creativity over the past forty years or so, transformed its institutions of governance and brought forth the first world order, more or less behind its own back.

This is a pretty rickety system, and any number of things may happen: It may collapse and take the biosphere with it. It may turn into a much more unified, even tyrannical, world government. It cannot, given the present inertial roll of globalizing forces, return to a system of autonomous nation-states. Neither can it, for the same set of reasons, sort itself out into a system of bioregional ecotopias. The latter is an attractive scenario, but not achievable this side of the population wave, since people have a tendency to move into your bioregion if they happen to be starving in their own. Nevertheless, the bioregional/ecotopian/small-is-beautiful approach has a great contribution to make: an interest in designing sub-systems that operate in such a way as to produce minimal externalities, pollutants, and impacts on their neighbors. The more such methods of growing food and producing goods and developing economies can be put into practice, the less need there will be for regulations and disaster relief projects. However, I doubt that bioregional ar-rangements will ever be quite as rural, benign, and au-tonomous as some of their proponents believe. The bior-gional urge is essentially an isolationist one, an attempt to buck the tide of global plant and animal transfer, and its proponents will find that protecting the integrity of a bioregion is as difficult as protecting the integrity of a race, a fundamentalist culture, or a sovereign nation.

I offer as a scenario for global governance in the short-term future a system that looks much like the one we have now: nation-states and intergovernmental organi-zations, multinational businesses and nongovernmental organizations, the whole apparatus being continually affected by globalizing forces, and continually modified by innovation under pressure. Acid pollution has already produced intense intergovernmental activity, especially in Europe, and could well become the focus of yet another intergovernmental organization. The promises of biotechnology cry out for new institutional forms. I expect many more Law of the Sea-type efforts to deal with large-scale problems of global governance, and more "two-track" or multiple-track arrangements of institutions, such as the proposed Enterprise company—much experimentation and diversity, with nation-states and multinational business continuing to have great power. In short, I expect a pattern of global governance somewhat similar to what I described earlier in this chapter as the pattern of nature: wheels within wheels, systems overlapping and interacting, systems of different sizes and different kinds, all of them changing in both cyclical and linear transitions.

The present global system has come into existence over the past forty years. In the next forty, it will face its greatest dangers and opportunites as the Biological Revolution unfolds and we begin to understand that governance is the management of a biosphere. The challenges can be met with a flexible and not altogether elegant system of global governance, and perhaps met more effectively than they could have been handled by the Parliament of Man. Such a loosely-coupled system can retain most of our institutions of governance, although I do not think it can retain some of our ideas about them: We can have nation-states, but we cannot have sovereignty in its historic form as a bellicose separateness from all external authority. That change can be made, partly because sovereignty is already more fiction than fact. Human institutions have always been adaptable. They go through amazing transitions: The Roman republic, enemy of monarchy, became the Roman Empire. Oppressor of Christianity, it brought forth the Roman Catholic Church and the Holy Roman Empire—which endured until it became, as many wits pointed out, neither holy nor Roman nor an empire. The United States of America may be destined to endure through similar metamorphoses. Even now it is not terribly united, its states are not states, and it is far less American than it used to be.

[8]

Creating a
Biopolitical Culture

WE KNOW that formal organizations such as nation-states and multinational corporations and intergovernmental bodies are not the sum total of a system of governance, any more than buildings are the sum total of a city. The real substance of a polis lies in its shared values and beliefs and myths and customs: its "habits of the heart," in Alexis de Tocqueville's phrase; its "common moral vocabulary," in the words of a recent study of American culture.[1] Political scientists have amply documented the striking differences between societies that have very similar constitutions but dissimilar "civic cultures." The political culture shows itself in the the things we do through political institutions and expect them to do for us, in the kinds of leaders we choose, and in the ideas we hold about the society's purposes and goals. Anthropologist Clyde Kluckhohn defined culture as, among other things, "a set of ready-made definitions of the situation which each participant only slightly retailors in his own idiomatic way."[2]

It is easy enough to define culture, difficult to say where it comes from. Some components of it are handed down from generation to generation, of course, and some are transferred laterally from one society to another. Culture is learned, and some of the psychological predispositions that shape culture are genetically inherited—but it is also created. New aspects of culture continually emerge, like mutants. And this is a central part of the evolutionary business at hand. Indeed, the great project in which we are all now engaged is more than anything else a matter of gaining a better understanding of cultural change itself, and bringing about a deliberate large-scale cultural transition in a relatively short period of time.

For the first time in history, it becomes possible to put the subject of culture on the table as an item of the human agenda, and to contemplate the creation of a civic culture appropriate to the human role in the biosphere. Stated this way, the subject sounds lofty and unapproachable, but in fact it is a very immediate business. Few of us get up close to the creation of international organizations, but culture-creating, in our modern mass-media world, is going on all around us. We are beginning to discover—many people are beginning to discover—that culture is something we do not merely passively inherit. This is a revolutionary discovery.

In Aristotle's time people were beginning to realize that institutions of governance were their own creations and that they could, through study and reasoning, discover some of the principles and create better political systems. Over the past few decades we have been reluctantly coming to understand that the human species, through its myriad interventions in the biosphere, also participates in the creation of the "natural" environment. With those first two

[276]

difficult ideas still only barely assimilated, we are moving to a third that may be the most difficult of all.

Human evolution has reached a point at which every person's relationship to his or her cultural heritage—the architecture of values and beliefs and myths and symbols that surrounds our lives and gives shape to our inner experience—has become fundamentally different from what it once was. The main feature of the change is a greater degree of choice. Membership in a culture is no longer an accident of birth and an immutable condition of one's lifetime. Many of us in the West move through subcultures almost as casually as we move through neighborhoods and relationships. We avoid knowing the full truth of this, and for good reason: Such choices engender much anxiety; a frightening freedom is revealed by any opportunity to choose what to believe, what to value, what sort of a heritage to claim allegiance to. But the situation, if comprehended, provides a part of the answer to how we may meet the challenges that lie just ahead, and it also offers a useful clue to what is happening now.

In this chapter we will deal with a matter which, although it lies at the very heart of the whole subject of evolutionary governance, is much less concrete than the material we have dealt with so far. It is possible to document the location of gene storage banks in the world, to count the number of children born through embryo transplant or artificial insemination, to keep track of the growth of intergovernmental organizations—but cultural change is a slippery subject. To make the going easier, I will set forth the chapter's central propositions, as I did in Chapter One regarding the book as a whole.

The first proposition is that a global culture is coming into being. This is not in itself a particularly daring assertion, since it is widely conceded to be true—even by people who wish it weren't—but it is fundamental to what follows.

The second is that we are in the midst of an evolution of cultural evolution, in which the conditions of cultural change are themselves changing. I will not be able to prove this (I am not at all sure it can be proved or disproved in any final way) but I will try to make clear what I mean by it and how it relates to the larger themes of this book.

The third is that the project of creating a global biopolitical culture is already underway—that many people have recognized both the reality of cultural globalism and the presence of a new set of rules of cultural change, and are trying to create values and beliefs appropriate to managing the biosphere.

The fourth is that some aspects of environmentalism provide some of the necessary elements of such a culture, but that it would be very naive to equate the values and beliefs of the environmental subculture that currently exists in the West with the global culture of the future.

The fifth, shifting from description to prescription, consists of some proposed basic elements of a biopolitical culture and a necessary course of action—an essential step toward the creation of a working biopolitical culture—that can be pursued both as public policy and as private initiative.

The Evolution of Cultural Evolution

IN ORDER to talk about this, we need to review some fundamentals of evolutionary theory.

The evolutionary biologists speak of two kinds of evolution: genetic, with information transmitted by DNA; and cultural, with information passed along through symbols. In the first, each of us has two parents and inherits enough information to make us acceptable company around a Stone Age campfire (although we would not know how to make the fire). In the second we have multiple parents and, depending on our intelligence, education, and social position, access to the expanding "gene pool" of human culture, everything in the world's brains and libraries and computer data banks.[3]

Global culture is a recent arrival. Like the artificial eco-systems in which we live, it pervades our lives but is scarcely noticed. If we think of it at all we are more likely to think of it as something "off there" than as something "in here," a part of our personal consciousness—but the world is very much with us. Some of us are more a part of world culture than others, but there remain few people whom it has not in some way touched. Its main vehicle is the mass media, and in part it merely appears to be a diffusion of Western popcult. But even that carries the implicit image of the world and a single human species. We know a global culture is emerging, yet its shape is hard to define.

I must admit that, although I am certain it is already here, I am not at all sure what it consists of—and I don't know of anybody who has undertaken to describe it. Science provides a part of it, and I have heard it persuasively argued that the view of the evolving cosmos presented now by the astronomers and physicists has the makings of a "new story" capable of uniting the species. Commerce is also a part of world culture; trade has always been a kind of universal language, and today, for better or for worse, the networks of international business gather us together into systems that require some agreed-upon ideas. But these are merely clues, rumors, shapes emerging from the mist. It is easier to get a clear image of global *sub*cultures like those of scientists and politicians: jet-setting international communities whose members share customs and jargon and are often more comfortable with one another than with their neighbors at home. These are indicators of a larger phenomenon. The emergence of a global culture—however amorphous, however stratified, however cluttered with T-shirts and rock music—is a major event in human evolution. It is not just a leap from the local but a much more compex reordering of social life. One study—whose title, *No Sense of Place*, summarizes its message of what electronic media do to the human sense of social space—describes a world with a "placeless" culture.[4] This produces a "homogenization of regional spheres" like the homogenization of ecosystems that is part of our new biological condition, and subcultures unbounded by geographic space. The analysis in some ways parallels my description of the global political system: It shows a multidimensional global culture that is not McLuhan's global village any more than the emerging polis is Tennyson's Parliament of Man—but is a system nonethless.

It is also a maxim of evolutionary biology that evolution evolves: Its rules change occasionally. The appearance of symbolic communication was one such event; it began human cultural evolution, and changed the rules for all living things. We are currently undergoing an evolution of *cultural* evolution, no less dramatic than the change of pace in *genetic* evolution manifest in rapid species extinction and the appearance of the new biotechnologies. It is not only a change, but a change in how culture changes.

There have been great cultural changes over the past few decades. We can't compare them precisely with similar changes at other times, since opinion sampling is itself one of the recent products of cultural evolution. We had no Gallup or Yankelovich to measure the shifts that occurred during the Renaissance or the French Revolution. But there is ample common-sense evidence that more people have modified their values and beliefs over the past few decades than over any other comparably brief period of time.

This is an awesome development, but yet only a symptom of a deeper transition that is taking place at the same time—a shift in the way we relate to culture itself. One aspect of this is an increasing degree of personal choice.

The conditions of contemporary life—the mobility, the explosion of information, the penetration of mass culture to all corners of the world, the political and economic upheavals—all conspire against the slow and orderly transmission of "cultural DNA" that perpetuates traditional societies. For most people since cultural evolution began, there was simply information to be acquired from others, and deeper kinds of knowledge, mythic or religious, to be absorbed through ritual and art. They had choices to make, but the range was narrow, and few had to trouble themselves about what lifestyle to adopt.

Even now, at this remarkable moment in history when old ways still remain even as the world plunges on into the unknown, one can find places where the absorbtion of culture is—or appears to be—simply a matter of taking in the truths accumulated by prior generations.

But for most of us, becoming socialized is a far more confusing business, demands a different kind of personal effort. We experience the usual pressures to conform—social demands from without, the instinctive drive from within—yet have a hard time finding out what it is we are to conform to. A bewildering range of subcultures spreads out before us like a smorgasbord, inviting each of us to choose what to value, what to believe, what kind of a person to be.

We have an array of subcultures, and much controversy about what is left of the larger national or Western culture that binds them together. It is hard to locate such a central structure at all. There is one—every society has a body of norms and information, values and beliefs that are shared by most of its members—but there is also a huge difference of opinion about what our cultural mainstream ought to contain. Since the 1960s, when cultural politics became the norm—with establishment pitted against counterculture—we have grown accustomed to a strange new mode of political conflict wherein polarization is not between classes or parties or even ideologies, but between contending cultures. And this cultural warfare is not just a matter of choosing lifestyles, deciding to dress or act in a certain way—although many took it to be little more than that—but a dialogue about how it is necessary for all people to be.

The cultural turmoil of our time reveals itself in different ways and produces different responses.

At one level it is just a condition of personal freedom. For many that freedom is delightful, the choices do not seem terribly important, and the whole thing is little more than a game. (In the 1960s Susan Sontag described the self-consciously whimsical game of "camp"; camp was, as she put it, an "aesthetic experience of the world," which "sees everything in quotation marks."[5]) Others find the freedom disturbing and take refuge in some more solid cultural environment that reduces options to a manageable number. One way is to make a voluntary adjustment of lifestyle to conform closely to tradition:

American Jews deciding to eat kosher and observe the rules of religious orthodoxy, for example. This is a kind of identity-affirmation most of us try at one time or another; it lets you take on as much tradition as you choose, an alternative not available in truly traditional societies where the usual choices were conformity or death. For those prepared to commit themselves to a more complete kind of mental environment, there is the cult, which provides in a single kit all the necessities of cultural security: leadership, values, beliefs, a cause greater than oneself, and a society of people who have bought the same package.

At another level are traditionalist movements like Islamic and Chrisian fundamentalism. Psychologically, these are identical to cults—motivated by the same needs, driven by the same internal dynamics. The chief difference is their greater ability to mobilize political power. Such movements are xenophobic, rigid, and desperately driven to maintain—by force if necessary—a social order in which all things are explained, all values clear and certain.

Fundamentalist movements do not consciously seek to create new cultural forms—although in fact that is what they do. Most claim a divine origin for their culture, and consequently are not open to the idea that there are new truths to be discovered, new values to be adopted, new myths to be brought to life.

But many people are convinced that something is to be created. The activists of this kind of cultural politics may be operating more or less as individuals—artists, scientists, philosophers—but more often we find them associated with movements.

The movement is the archetypal political phenomenon of the second half of the twentieth century. The word "movement" itself is promiscuously applied, which signals that something is going on that doesn't quite fit the vocabulary. Some, such as the black movement and the women's movement, conform to our notion of what a movement should be: They represent identifiable interest groups and have tangible political goals. Others, such as the hippie movement, the human potential movement, the drug movement, are hard to categorize. Some are quite uninterested in public policy; some are scarcely aware of it.

But there is a common feature of the modern movement: its desire to influence cultural change. Not all movements are playing politics as we have known it, but all are playing culture—seeking to modify the transmission of consciousness; to influence how people behave, what they value and believe to be true.

The appearance of such movements results from the discovery that culture is itself an artifact, something to be changed or discarded, cherished or created. That discovery is the pivotal point of the evolution of evolution that is occurring in our time.

Julian Huxley spoke of evolution becoming conscious of itself; however, the event he described—the publication of Darwin's theory—was only cultural evolution becoming conscious of genetic evolution. Now cultural evolution is becoming conscious of cultural evolution. This is a shift in perspective, rather like the one visually symbolized by the photograph of the Earth, in which something familiar is seen in a breathtakingly new way. New choices and new problems emerge. People begin to talk about what kind of myths we need—a subject that would have been literally unthinkable in earlier times—and the stage is set for the entry of all the phenomena of contemporary life: cults and deprogrammers, fundamentalists and fascists, punks and anarchists, alienation and identity crises, cultural anthropologists studying myths and belief systems, poets lamenting that the centre cannot hold. A thin wedge is driven between society and consciousness in every mind, an unruly element of personal volition intrudes, and we enter a new world in which yet another part of the edifice of reality is built by human hands. This change promises to be—like the appearance of symbolic communication itself—a whole-system change that will affect all life on Earth.

Green Culture

OF ALL the movements and counter-movements of our time, the most clearly evolutionary is environmentalism. It has begun the first global dialogue about human intervention in nature.

It is in that respect our most important movement, and also the most imperfect; imperfect in the sense of being unfinished. Environmentalism is so many-sided that in some ways it is best compared to broad shifts in the *zeitgeist* like the Romantic Movement. It is neither conspiracy nor cult nor organization. It has organizations of all shapes and sizes, but you don't have to join one to become a part of it.

Environmentalism is a subculture, a global political movement and a religious movement—in the third respect, more successful than the churches at getting religious issues into the mainstream of public dialogue. Despite the maxim that politics and religion don't mix (one of our most relentlessly violated cultural norms anyway) environmentalism has mixed the two rather well, and since its appearance in the United States it has managed to move

American culture some distance along both the secular and the spiritual tracks.

When environmentalism came on the American scene around 1970, it looked like a familiar species of domestic political life—the reform movement. Like the good-government binge of some decades before, it was preceded by an escort of muckrakers. Rachel Carson's *Silent Spring* performed the same function that the works of Ida Tarbell and Lincoln Steffens and Upton Sinclair had done for the earlier movement. Environmentalism also started from the same demographic base. Its cadre had roots in the old conservationism and was largely white, prosperous, and educated.

The environmental muckrakers showed that the system was not working as it should, and the response was a search for remedies—reform legislation, preferably at the federal level.

Many laws were passed and in some ways conditions improved, yet somewhere along the line it became apparent that the environmental cause was not a minor malfunction to be repaired by a few adjustments in public policy. It was something much larger than that.

There was a hint of this in the curious ripples that it raised on the political Left. The movement when it appeared had seemed so clearly another liberal cause, with powerful new ammunition to use against big business, that it was hard to believe it would not find favor with other liberal causes. But it annoyed some leaders of racial minority movements, and totally failed to win the hearts of organized labor. It was not the first new cause to have such an effect on the unions—the anti-Vietnam war movement had touched this same conservative nerve—but it created serious conflict between labor and other liberal groups, united

[286]

labor and management in many battles over development projects, and thus showed an ability to alter old polarizations of American political life that could hardly be expected of some passing elitist fad.

Environmentalism mounted a major critique of the Industrial Revolution, as far-reaching as Marxism but—lacking its Marx and its Manifesto—slower to communicate its revolutionary intent. Marxists had complained about how the rewards of industry were divided; environmentalists complained about what industry *did*, charged that it was poisoning the air and water and the workers at the same time. Marxism had been a pure theory of conflict that located evil in the ruling class; environmentalism handed down a more sweeping indictment that found some measure of wrongdoing in everybody—some flaw in the way we all live. One of its most-quoted slogans was the line from the Pogo comic strip: "We have met the enemy and he is us."

Environmentalists wanted people to live differently. It was not enough to contribute a few dollars, vote for right-thinking candidates; you were expected to show a greater concern for your own impact upon the world. Recycle your garbage. Put a brick in your water closet. When the energy crisis arrived, environmental consciousness became something to be expressed in insulating your home, going solar, riding a bicycle, driving a smaller car. A whole mystique of frugal living developed, strikingly different from American consumerism in which extravagance was practically a civic virtue. It was not a total departure from American cultural tradition—Thoreau's memory was often invoked—but neither was it in the shopping-plaza mainstream. It was always talking about the whole Earth, and it offered both a new value system and an answer to the problem of political participation and personal power-lessness: It insisted that everyone could do something, merely by rearranging the operations of daily life.

For many people this can be addressed in secular terms and restricted to matters of self-interest: Energy conservation saves money, organic gardening produces healthful food. But the secular veneer is thin. Scratch a solar energy expert and you find a mystic. Start a conversation about digging in the dirt, and you end up talking about meditation.

When the new environmental movement arrived—floating, like all information-era phenomena, on a tidal wave of literature—it included a surprising sprinkling of theology. One of the essays commonly found in the collections of environmental thought was Lynn White Jr.'s "The Historical Roots of our Ecologic Crisis," which called Christianity "the most anthropocentric religion the world has seen," and charged that it "not only established a dualism of man and nature but also insisted that it is God's will that man exploit nature for his proper ends."[6] White's protest set off a round of theological discussion. White thought highly of St. Francis of Assisi, and proposed him as the "patron saint of ecologists," model for a new vision of the human role, based more on a passive appreciation of its wonders. This view found much favor among environmentalists, but René Dubos challenged what he called its "romantic and unworldly" belief that humanity was ever merely a "passive witness of his surroundings and natural events." Dubos proposed an alternature culture hero, Benedict of Nursia, and commended the Benedictine model of creative stewardship, visible, he said, in "its wisdom in managing the land, in fitting architecture to worship and landscape, in adapting rituals and work to cosmic rhythms."[7]

Those two points of view set up a still-ongoing debate about eco-theology. Alan Watts' essay, "The Individual as Man/World" (another environmental classic) offered a third point of view that sought to transcend the controversy. Watts took issue with the idea that there was any human reality truly separate from nature; he argued for a conception of the individual "not, on the one hand, as an ego locked in the skin, nor, on the other, as a mere passive part of the machine, but as a reciprocal interaction between everything inside the skin and everything outside it, neither one being prior to the other, but equals, like the front and back of a coin."[8]

Watts' work, like so much of what has become part of the environmental culture, derives from Eastern religion. No other political movement has drawn so heavily on non-Western religious sources. The chapter on "Buddhist economics" in E.F. Schumacher's *Small Is Beautiful* is another work in which Western society's growing interest in Eastern culture—which some historians see as one of the most significant developments of the century—coincides with the search for new perspectives on humanity and nature.[9]

Another source of eco-theology is American Indian lore. Many environmentalists believe that pre-Columbian cultures showed a higher reverence for the natural world, and seek to bring that reverence back into American life. This is a worthy cause, and at the same time it illustrates some of the perils of shopping for religions and one of the weaknesses of the contemporary environmental mystique. We are profoundly in need of a more reverent mood toward the great enterprise of which we are a part, and we would all do well to study and understand the destructiveness that accompanied the conquest of the American continent. But we cannot simply transplant the consciousness of the people of one culture into our own—especially when we do not know what that consciousness was, nor live in the environment that gave birth to it. Culture-creating is naturally eclectic, and there is always the danger that in seeking to honor the values and beliefs of another people we project our own wishes upon them, and retreat again, as people so often have in challenging times, into comforting fantasies of the Golden Age of the past. The modern white Americans who seek to recapture the tradition of those cultures would do well to heed a theologian's recent reminder that, whereas tradition is the living faith of the dead, traditionalism is the dead faith of the living.[10]

Environmentalism has become far more than another reform movement. It has produced a body of political thought, and blown fresh ideas into the rather stagnant air of Western theology. It has unleashed a full range of forces for cultural change, everything from scientific information about environmental conditions to new mythic and symbolic images. Many of the images have to do with reverence for the Earth: We hear of the Greeks' Earth goddess Gaia, and are repeatedly exposed to what may be the key visual image of the emerging global culture, the astronauts' haunting blue photograph of the Earth, the whole Earth.

The public opinion polls report a high level of support for environmental goals. Political scientist Lester Milbrath concludes from the findings of one survey project: "The public is fairly aware that certain technological developments, production processes, and waste disposal practices have the potential to inflict injury on innocent people. They support regulations and procedures to insure that these activities do not place people at undue risk. Most people have begun to recognize that there are resource shortages, that limits must be placed on population growth, that we must learn to conserve rather than blindly rush to produce and consume, and that there are limits to growth."[11]

However, Pollyanna herself would not say that environmentalist attitudes have conquered Western culture, and there remains the more serious question of whether our problems would all be solved if they did. Milbrath's study holds that the cultural crisis of our time is easily resolved as soon as the "New Environmental Paradigm" sweeps away the prevailing value and belief structure. But in the process of stating the problem in such terms it overdraws the contrast between environmental virtue and an otherwise sinful world. Environmentalists, it asserts, "value nature for its own sake," and many of them "have an almost worshipful love of it." The environmentalists' value system is contrasted to that of "a society that uses nature to produce the goods we use."[12] This facile dichotomization avoids any discussion of what nature is, and does not tell us how the people who qualified as environmentalists managed not to use nature to produce their goods. The researchers clearly invited people to respond to survey questions on a merely rhetorical basis, and the resultant study makes a difficult cultural transition seem a good deal neater than it will ever be.

Stumbling toward Biopolitics

THE ENVIRONMENTAL movement, for all its complexity, is really only a curtain-raiser.

The human species is stepping forth—perhaps stumbling is the better word—onto a larger stage in which every act has impacts and implications we did not heretofore suspect. We find that since before recorded history our ancestors have been intervening in evolution, and that they have left us a world which is in many ways strikingly unimproved by their efforts—yet we do not know how to undo their interventions, nor do we know how to stop intervening ourselves. We have an idea of evolution that is not very old as ideas go and scarcely assimilated into our belief system—still challenged, in fact, by brigades of grumpy creationists. While we fight rear-guard actions over the idea of evolution, our impact upon it increases with each child born, with every working day in the laboratories, with every hectare of tropical forest that falls before the axe.

This is a concern of public policy; and, as we have seen, there are many agencies of government already dealing with evolutionary issues and many more just getting into the act. It will call for the creation of new institutional arrangements; and we see signs of that as well. And we need something that runs deeper, gives form to governance and provides some framework for people to agree and disagree: a political culture suited for a species that is becoming aware of its evolutionary role.

A strict Burkean or a contemporary scholar of political culture, noting how little in our heritage speaks to that issue, would not be sanguine about our prospects for moving into an era of evolutionary governance. But here we are nonetheless, and we are obliged to assemble about ourselves a structure of values and beliefs, norms and information, myths and symbols appropriate to the tasks at hand. The culture-creating which has become such a familiar and often entertaining feature of modern life stands revealed as a matter of fierce importance to the future of the human species and to all the other life-forms whose evolutionary destinies are linked to our own.

How will we recognize a biopolitical culture when it does in fact begin to emerge among us? What will we be arguing about, worrying about, hoping for? What values will we cherish, what will we believe to be true? What mythic images will shape our feelings and thoughts? I would not pretend to be able to paint a picture in detail, but there are certain elements that the conditions of the time render necessary.

Among these, certainly, are some of the values and beliefs that have been championed by the environmental movement—such as a sense of the importance of the biosphere's well-being and a willingness to adjust the habits of personal life to serve that need—but I do not think the future is entirely in the keeping of the environmentalists.

Consider, as a way of approaching this subject, Ernest Callenbach's novel *Ecotopia*: The Ecotopians, with cheerful unity of purpose, conserve energy, recycle materials, ride public transportation, grow organic food, and support their political leaders—mostly women—in running a "stable state" system.[13] *Ecotopia* gives a picture of what a society with a strongly environmentalist value system might look like, and it also gives a point of departure; it suggests where an environmental ethic leaves off and a biopolitical one begins.

First of all, Ecotopia is isolated from the rest of the world—a necessary convention of the utopian novel, but a biopolitical impossibility. The Ecotopians are reverent and caring toward their part of the planet, and they do no harm to the world beyond their boundaries: They do not plunder its resources, crowd into it with their surplus population, throw smoke into its atmosphere, dump untreated effluent into its seas, or sell toxic chemicals to its farmers. On the other hand, they seem immune to its problems. Acid rain does not fall on Ecotopia. The country does not have to do anything about world population. No fruit flies or exotic diseases cross its boundaries. Its gene banks are presumably well-stocked and in need of no seeds from elsewhere in the world. The Ecotopians are responsible stewards of the land, but they are convinced separatists and localists—not members of the global polis.

Ecotopia speaks more from the bioregional perspective of environmentalism than for the the global message of the movement. A biopolitical culture will have to absorb the global message, and go well beyond it. The citizens of societies in the years just ahead of us will have to be— to a degree that people have never been before—citizens of the world. And this will be a practical business. If people in individualistic and isolationist America, and people struggling for survival in Third World countries, are to become global citizens it will have to come about in large part because they know that their lives truly are parts of a global system, and not merely because they have been converted to vague sentiments of global unity. The global polis will probably be full of conflict, and I suspect the global culture will contain a great range of subcultural diversity and fervent separatist ideologies. But a political culture in which people *know* they inhabit the biosphere will also generate new ideologies and programs of global interaction.

Ecotopia is a stable social system, with a high degree of political consensus, a tranquil economy, and a biological infrastructure that is not plunging through the genetic rapids. Its citizens seem to have arrived at where they had wanted to go. Again, this is a necessary result of the utopian novelist's job—which is to show a desirable society—but it points to something that will *not* be a part of our political culture in the decades ahead. We will know that we live in a world that is changing, even changing the way it changes, and we will understand our lives and societes in those terms.

Where the Ecotopians had their value systems pretty well figured out, we will be required to examine and continually modify ours. The postmodern era will seek not only scientific truths but ethical principles. In the modern era, morality receded into the background. Even though many people were deeply concerned about moral issues, the political culture as a whole subordinated that to its belief that politics is a clash of interests rather than ideals and that the effective politician is a "pragmatist"— a word which, in American usage, has come to connote a Machiavellian power broker who never lets principles clutter up the deal. This is the culture that gave birth to "value-free" research in the social sciences, and to Daniel Bell's premature announcement of the "end of ideology."

The coming age is foreshadowed in the growing field of "bioethics", in the presence of ethical specialists on hospital staffs, in the discourse about animal rights, in the existence of think tanks such as the Hastings Center in New York—originally named the Institute of Society, Ethics and the Life Sciences. Organized religion may provide the institutional setting for much of this ongoing dialogue. The churches, rooted in everyday family and community life, could be the ideal places for people to grapple with the issues of a postmodern world at a grass-roots level. However, if the churches do take on such a role, they will themselves be changed by it and not merely be agents of change. A search for ethical responses to the new conditions of life can be productive only when those who would act as guides are themselves well-informed about precisely what these conditions are. If the churches are to serve as an ethical forum for the Biological Revolution, clergy of the future are going to have to plunge into ecological and biological education the way clergy of recent decades have educated themselves about psychology in order to serve as counsellors. Uninformed homilies about stewardship will not do the job.

The women's movement is another contemporary development that has the potential of becoming a major force in global political culture—and, again, not quite in the way that is envisioned by environmentalists. There is an "eco-feminist" school of thought within the environmental mystique that holds women to be inherently in possession of a superior ecological wisdom, and I see no evidence whatever that this is true. My vision may be clouded by memories of Ann Gorsuch Burford. However, women must be full members of the global polis and have a claim to be heard in a special way about what it becomes. The women's movement began its own Biological Revolution by questioning the link between sex and social role. And it is inseparable from the other Biological Revolution that we identify with scientific discoveries and technological change. For example, new methods of birth control give women—at least, women in the developed nations—an unprecedented ability to make choices about their reproductive lives, and a corresponding ability to choose social roles other than those of wife and mother. As similar choices and the ideas that go with them become available to women in other regions of the world, we may see that the Biological Revolution is truly revolutionary. As our organic lives change, inevitably the practice of basing social roles on biological functions comes into question. The widely divergent positions taken by feminists in regard to the new reproductive technologies can be regarded, then, as overtures to a far-reaching political process whereby women assert their particular interest in shaping public policies in this area. This will be a major cultural shift, and it can best be comprehended not by imagining what will be its ultimate product, but by recognizing that a civic culture is definable by what it is dealing with. And a society engaged in such a dialogue is different from any we have known in the modern world.

We commonly describe cultures by their answers, but the best way to approach the subject of a biopolitical culture is by its questions. This is also the best way to identify its difference from environmentalism. Environmentalists tend to take the position that modern society has had the wrong answer about the humanity/nature interface and environmentalism offers the right one. I don't think so. I think, rather, that the global culture which will be the reality of our near-term future will be one in which people everywhere are intensely living in the questions—engaged in a life-and-death search for understanding about our place in the biosphere. This will be both a search for information and a search for meaning; it will involve religion and science, psychology and politics. And for some time to come the questions themselves will be our new habits of the heart.

In order to ask the right questions we must have a good sense of what is already known. We have available a great deal more good knowledge about how matters currently stand with humanity and the biosphere than we are using, and we must do everything possible to bring that knowledge into the mainstream of our personal lives and public dialogue.

Getting Here

A SOCIETY develops a common moral vocabulary out of common perceptions about what is going on in its world. Cultural values rest on a base of information. This gives us an opening to consider what can reasonably be done—how we might cease stumbling toward biopolitics and move toward it more purposefully—because there is a serious deficiency of information in contemporary society.

This seems a curious thing to say in the midst of the Information Revolution—and to say of a society that may well be the best-informed the world has ever seen. But despite the proliferation of data about our environment and the increasing currency of concepts of the biosphere, despite the presence of public and private bodies totally devoted to producing such information, we are not a biologically literate people; our knowledge of the realities of our organic existence is in no way equal to the need to make decisions about it, either as individuals or as citizens.

We do not have a deep feeling for our present condition—we do not really know where *here* is—and when you don't know where you are you are not in a brilliant position to discuss where to go next. The way to create a political culture that can chart out an evolutionary future is to get a better idea of the evolutionary present. I have always been attracted to the gestalt therapists' proposition that agendas for personal change are continually stifled by weak awareness of what is happening in the here and

[298]

now, and that you cannot set out on a new personal path until you come to terms with what you are currently doing.

Although environmentalism and environmental education are firmly established in public policy, most of us do not know much about what we do to the environment, and we know still less about what it does to us. We are educated in history, but less sure of natural history. Americans (both North and South) know little about the long sequence of events whereby the New World was remodeled for their convenience, and are not really prepared to exercise responsible citizenship about how that rebuilt hemisphere should be managed and used now.

There is a similar lack of working wisdom about the public life support systems which we depend upon and yet casually take for granted. Few people know where their water comes from, other than out of a tap, or where it goes, other than down the drain. This is fine as long as the systems are functioning smoothly at both ends, but it shows where the sense of personal boundaries lies, and reveals how shaky is the base from which we try to understand our relationship to nature and to political systems.

In California, in the early years of this century, there was a classic conflict between what were then the two main wings of the American conservation movement: preservationists and utilitarians. The subject of this controversy was a proposal to build a dam in the beautiful Hetch Hetchy valley of Yosemite, and bring water from it to San Francisco. John Muir, founder of the Sierra Club and leader of the preservationists, fought to save the Hetch Hetchy. Other conservationists (this was a true civil war) advocated taking the water, and became known as the utilitarians. The utilitarians won, and the dam was built. So were other dams, and all of us who live in this region are organically a part of the water system that has resulted.

And I have been present at gatherings where people whose hearts pumped blood manufactured from the waters of the High Sierra—and who thereby qualified as *de facto* utilitarians—spoke of how they had learned from the study of Buddhism that the human race should not interfere with nature, and mentioned also, in a kind of satisfied way, that they were not much into politics.

They literally did not know how their bodies were kept alive.

The problem here is not hypocrisy, but something more subtle which is a major obstacle to any effort to build a new culture suitable to our biological responsibilities. It is a sort of cultivated ignorance about the present realities of our organic existence. Something is not known: even if known as information, not known as bone-deep experience. We have an idea of ecosystems, but not of noosystems. Our minds remain in the Garden even when our bodies are here in the world created by *Homo intervenor*.

Surely the problem is not inability to absorb information. Consider the incredible amounts of environmental lore known to some primitive societies—such as the seagoing peoples of Polynesia—or the modern person's knowledge of the intricacies of the economic system: We follow the economic news with the same avid interest with which people of another society might have observed the changes of the seasons or the movements of game animals. Ups and downs of the stock market, of interest rates, of the exchange value of the dollar, are front-page news. Every educated person holds views on the relationships among these statistics; pundits of the mass media and candidates for high office seize on any opportunity to display their economic wisdom.

A moment's contemplation of our national obsession with the minutae of economic life affords us an excellent oportunity to get a look at ourselves, as if in a mirror, and to imagine what a society might be like if its members were as serious about the biological side of life as we are about the economic. The front pages would give the latest news on genetic diversity, the TV news would keep us informed about the health of ecosystems, no politician would run for office without a biologist or two as top advisers, the people would cheer a president who could boast that the rate of species extinction had not risen during his years in office, and competing parties would offer different approaches to global ecological management.

There is a way to move in that direction, and it has to do with something well within the scope of public policy: education. Our history has many precedents for programs of deliberate cultural evolution. When, in the early years of this century, Americans feared an erosion of our cultural heritage as the immigrants poured in, the government launched an "Americanization" program to teach new-comers about our history and political institutions, expose them to new values, and inspire them with the myths and symbols of democracy. Later, when the country believed itself threatened by Soviet superiority in space, the federal government moved speedily to improve the quality of education in the appropriate fields of science—declared it in the public interest that the United States produce a new generation of space scientists.

A national program to raise the level of public awareness of biopolitical matters and issues would educate about the matrix of relationships in which life is sustained: the actions

[301]

and public agencies which oversee the air we breathe and the water we drink, the systems which provide our food, the questions and concerns about toxic chemicals and health, the issues concerning species extinction and genetic erosion and priority-setting in genetic technology, the changing conditions of human reproduction. The aim would be— as the Americanization program sought to turn subjects of European monarchies into informed participants in a democracy, and the space program sought to educate for the space age—to produce well-informed citizens of a biopolitical age, and a generation of scientists of ecology and life. And although such an educational program would undoubtedly be richly seasoned with new biological knowledge, it would not make sense unless there were also a solid grounding in history: "natural" history, the record of evolution including the record of human in-volvement in it. The scope would, of course, have to be global as well, so that the kind of information currently accumulating about global conditions—and so far the province of a relatively limited audience of fretful Earth-watchers—might become as public as the news of who won the last Super Bowl.

Up to a point, the kind of educational effort I am proposing fits rather neatly within the boundaries of political possibility. Up to a point. It is fairly non-controversial as long as the proposal is to teach facts—but the essence of the Biological Revolution is to bring us facts that are by no means value-free; they cry out to be interpreted, to be humanized with meaning and choice. The matter becomes even more politically touchy when it begins to deal explicitly with evolution—a subject which is itself a matter of anguished controversy, one of the most heated issues of contemporary educational politics.

And some will call education for global citizenship a subversion of patriotic values. We will see a revival of the dialogue that America's most revered philosopher of education, John Dewey, was engaged in decades ago when he insisted that the "social aim" of education was to produce citizens who were responsible members of the human species. Dewey (another man who was ahead of his time) said that the social aim was not to be confused with or subordinated to a national aim.

There is no way around these conflicts, and there should not be a way around them. Differences, if clearly stated and engaged by those who hold opinions, are one of our best vehicles of cultural change.

The controversy about whether the human race should dominate nature or leave it alone—which threads through so much of the public discussion of the matters discussed in this book, and which is implicit in studies such as Milbrath's public-opinion research—is one in which it is much easier to hold extreme positions as long as one has not delved too deeply into the realities of how the human/ nature system really works.

As one does explore those realities one is taken into a worldview that is somewhere beyond that polarization, something closer to Alan Watts's vision. In that frame of reference there are still problems of monumental difficulty and plenty to argue about—but the arguments are likely to be much more productive.

Nature lovers often counsel—wisely—that everyone take the time to become acquainted with the ecosystem in which he or she lives: learn something of its native flora and fauna, understand its geology and its weather patterns. I suggest that the person who would be an active citizen of our time do that and extend the inquiry also to the non-native life and the artificial systems. As we do we understand that our ecosystem is the world, and is also the political system and the cultures which we inhabit and which inhabit us—and perhaps we come to understand also that they are all of a seamless whole: We can see that there is no nature if we look long and hard at the evidence of human intervention, or we can flip the coin, consider that human intelligence is but another of evolution's many odd inventions, and see that there is no non-nature.

This discovery is one that can be made by each of us. It can be learned and it can be taught, and it also can be made a part of our public philosophy, a web to bind together the many elements of a new polis.

Learning and Governing

WE NEED not only adult education for a new kind of citizenship and a new kind of education in the schools and publicly supported scientific research but also a larger frame of reference that embraces them all. We need to become a society actively engaged in the business of learning. We need a value system—a public philosophy, a common moral vocabulary—which defines the good society as one that makes social learning its highest priority, knows something of how to go about it, and understands the centrality of learning to governance.

Education, so highly rated (if not always highly supported) in American society, is the best context in which to see how evolution and governance come together. We know that we have impacts upon the global environment and other living things, we see that when we find out what those impacts are we change what we do, and we naturally seek to know more—especially as we discover that the environment which we alter turns around and alters us. The *kubernetes* concept is essentially an ethic of learning.

We have noted, in the foregoing chapters, some of the adventures the political animal now confronts. Each of these involves learning—and not only learning, but learning about learning.

A conventional response to the challenge of evolutionary governance—that is, a response not informed by an ethic of learning—would assume that the thing to do is sit down and plan out where evolution goes from here. That is precisely what we cannot do. We cannot chart out a neat action plan of the sort that bureaucracies fancy, because we do not know enough. Neither can we set in motion a huge research program and sit back and wait for the results before we act, because we are acting every moment. Instead we act and learn, learn about the actions already performed, set real goals even while knowing they may change, and adjust course regularly.

The new political culture will have to be based on a learning mode of governance, involving constant processing of information and regular adjustments of course. This is going to come hard to autocratic governments guided by the myth of the all-knowing leader. We need, for entry into an age of evolutionary governance, a model of leaders as good learners, of planning as a learning process, and of good governance as an activity in which uncertainty goes with being well-informed, where mistakes are expected, and where changes of policy (sometimes major ones) are seen as signs of strength instead of weakness.[14]

I realize that my talk of culture-creating will seem to many readers to disregard the arguments of the socio-bioligists (and their precedessors) that the forms of society

[305]

are to some extent determined by the genes. But the scope of cultural creativity is not reduced by the reminder that we have social instincts, any more than the stature of the human species was reduced by the Darwinian message that we are blood relatives of the rest of earthly life. We did not become more apelike by discovering evolution, and we do not become more captives of our instincts by learning that we have them.

No pure genetic determinism for the social behavior of human adults has ever been proven, in any case. The sociobiologists reveal many fascinating analogies between human and animal societies, but none of those add up to scientific proof that any specific human social form or action is mandated by genetic information alone.[15] The best that can be said for the sociobiological case is that it reveals certain potentials: a "tangled wing", in the phrase of one of the best available books on the subject, in which instinct and culture overlap and interact.[16] War, as the general systems theorist Ludwig von Bertalanffy once pointed out, is made possible by the fact that human beings are genetically capable of intra-specific aggression—made possible, but not inevitable. Human warfare itself is not reducible to genetic determinism, but requires an elaborate symbolic framework of abstractions and ideology.[17] So if we accept the hypothesis that there is some genetic basis for most human behaviors, we are not driven, as some of sociobiology's opponents seem to fear, into dour acceptance of the inevitability of aggression, authoritarianism, hierarchy and patriarchy. We have information, uncertainty, and choices.

For example: Some sociobiologists theorize that humans are genetically better suited to face-to-face interactions in small groups and that small-scale participatory democracy is thus inherently superior to large and impersonal bureaucratic systems.[18] This proposition is not proven, and we can accept it or reject it. If we accept it, it becomes the basis of a system of values and beliefs and we have a wide range of creative possibilities for applying it; we can even (remembering that there are social institutions such as ritual suicide and celibacy that override the strongest instincts) create systems that deliberately thwart the drive.

Sociobiology itself—its insights, its limitations, the political and ethical arguments it raises—becomes a part of our culture, something else to learn about, and does not by any means provide programmed answers to the questions that open up as we explore the freedoms and responsibilities of the human condition. It does not take away our self-creativity, but only gives a new dimension and a twentieth-century meaning to Pico della Mirandola's famous Renaissance oration in which he has God say to Adam that "you, being your own free maker and artificer, may fashion yourself into whatever form you choose."[19] The options today are infinitely greater, and today God would also say the same thing to Eve.

[9]

Politics on a New Scale: Dangers and Opportunities

THE EVENTS of the modern era have fundamentally restructured the conditions of human personal and social existence. Throughout this turbulent moment of evolutionary history (whose beginning I arbitrarily marked with Turgot's speech on the inevitability of human progress) there has been a steady line of movement—not, as Turgot and the other apostles of progress believed, constant betterment of the human condition, but rather constant increase of human intervention in the workings of the biosphere. There has also been a steady and not always welcome increase in the development of feedback mechanisms that enable (or force) us to know the consequences of our interventions and show how much of the world we live in is of our own making. More power, and more knowledge. This power and knowledge are carrying us into a postmodern world in which the scale of politics, the basic parameters of political space and time, are different from what we have known in the very recent past. The spacial framework is the whole Earth; the time dimension seems to be understandable only in terms of exponential change.

The authors of *GAIA: An Atlas of Planet Management* offer this arresting summary of the evolutionary time scale:

> Throughout its 15 billion years, the pace of the universe's development has been accelerating, each new wave of innovation building up to trigger the next, in a series of "leaps" up to further levels of diversification and change. Compress this unimaginable timescale into a single 24-hour day, and the Big Bang is over in less than a ten-billionth of a second. Stable atoms form in about four seconds; but not for several hours, until early dawn, do stars and galaxies form. Our own solar system must wait for early evening, around 6 p.m. Life on Earth begins around 8 p.m., the first vertebrates crawl on to land at about 10:30 at night. Dinosaurs roam from 11:35 p.m. until four minutes to midnight. Our ancestors first walk upright with ten seconds to go. The Industrial Revolution, and all our modern age, occupy less than the last thousandth of a second. Yet in this fraction of time, the face of this planet has changed almost as much as in all the aeons before.[1]

This suggests that exponential change is not just something to be found in certain human affairs, but is a phenomenon of the evolution of the cosmos. We really don't know that much about the cosmic time scale, but we do have ample evidence of the changing pace of evolution on this planet, and there is every reason to believe that human power to intervene in the workings of the biosphere will not only continue to increase, but will increase at accelerating speed for some time to come. Some of the exponential changes that have been set in motion by our interventions—such as the loss of species and the growth of human population—will have to level off. But if they do so it will be because we have begun to practice other kinds of intervention; the master curve, the rise in human power and knowledge, promises to continue upward.

In view of the monumental number of problems we have already, this is a rather intimidating prospect. If we recall that the appearance of a theory of evolution—bringing the news that the order of life on Earth was not fixed and stable, but changing—had a "convulsing" effect on society, then the general recognition that the rate of change is something far greater than anyone in Darwin's time suspected may well prove to be even more disturbing. We are looking at the prospect of decades of rapid changes in the biosphere, and of corresponding upheavals in politics, economics, culture and personal life. I am often reminded these days that the Chinese ideogram for "crisis" is a combination of the signs for "danger" and "opportunity". That has become something of a cliche, in fact, but it may be a cliche worth heeding as we try to comprehend where we are and where we can go from here.

The Escalation of Intentionality

GROWING ABILITY to intervene in nature coupled with more knowledge about the effects of intervention produce not only a change in dimensions—toward globalism and exponential change—but also a greater degree of what the existential philosophers call intentionality. As more of life on earth is touched by human activity, more of the things that people do are infused with conscious choice, awareness of consequences.

This affects every individual, relationship, and organization. It produces options and possibilities, and also stress and confusion and resistance. Even though humanity has striven with unswerving purpose to win power and knowledge, we are rudely astonished to find that we have them—and even more astonished to find that they have us. I am reminded of the saying that you should be careful about what you want, because you might end up getting it.

Power and knowledge saturate our existence—private and public, local and global, cradle and grave. Mating couples steer their romantic lives through the intricacies of birth control, amniocentesis, genetic screening and counseling, artificial insemination, *in vitro* fertilization and surrogate motherhood, while pro-lifers and pro-choicers do battle over the morality of such decisions and scientists labor to create still more power over the reproductive process, to encumber prospective parents with more choices and more information. At the other end of the human lifespan, people come to death meeting all the ancient stresses of that occasion plus a whole new set of concerns about how and how long to be kept alive. Their last moments are crowded not only with hope and fear of the hereafter, memories and regrets of the past, but decisions about the life-support system. Out of this comes one more biopolitical crusade: Marching along in the opposite direction from those who make their cause the right to life, another movement champions the right to die.

Between birth and death, our lives are enormously different from those of our ancestors—people genetically no different from ourselves. Our veins flow with resistance against disease. Our teeth are repaired and our eyes bespectacled. Some of us have artificial joints and prosthetic limbs; some of us live by daily doses of insulin from other animals or from genetic engineering; some of us live in connection with kidney dialysis machines; some of us have pacemakers, even transplanted hearts. Our food is grown here and there about the world: Take a sip of coffee and you link your nervous system to the economies and ecosystems of distant countries; read a newspaper and you cannot avoid information about what is in your food, what it does to you and what you, by consuming it, do to the land where it is grown or to the animals from whom it is made. We must make choices about our social relationships, religions, political identities, lifestyles. We are asked to take care about how much energy we use, how much waste we produce, how many children we have, in the interest of some ecological public interest that few had heard of a few decades ago.

Organizations have similar problems. Industries that happily dumped their effluents into the air and water are now told they shouldn't do that—confronted with evidence of the effects of pollution on local water systems, on the land, on the air, on distant lakes, on the workers, on people who live nearby. Economists have introduced a new word into the political vocabulary: externalization. The concept, which became a major environmentalist weapon, holds that a certain segment of the cost of production bypasses the price system and is handed over to the public in pollution cleanup costs, public health expenses, and the like.[2] The externalization critique reveals that industry is exercising a power not previously a part of its reckoning—intervening in ecosystems and in the organic lives of plants, animals, human beings. This is a power that industry did not want to know it had, and much less for the public to know it had. The discovery changes the social context of industrial production. Managers come to terms with it in various ways: by cleaning up pollution, by going into the business of manufacturing products to clean up pollution, by getting the government to clean up pollution, by running institutional advertisements to proclaim their environmental goodness, by locating plants in places where the pollution laws are nonexistent or languidly enforced. There are many ways to play; the important thing to understand is that it is a new industrial ballgame.

Institutions of government also take on new power and new knowledge. The environmentalism of the 1960s and 1970s produced, predictably enough, new federal legislation: the National Environmental Policy Act, the Endangered Species Act, the clean air and water laws, later the Toxic Substances Control Act. This created additional powers— and a sector of government which continues to increase— yet it became apparent early on that government was problem as well as solution. Federal agencies like the Corps of Engineers became leading environmental heavies as people questioned their authority to remold the continent. Farther down the public hierarchy, cities emerged as great water polluters, rivaling the worst industries in some parts of the country.

In government as in industry, we find a previously unnoticed class of impacts: not merely environmental impacts, which are trouble enough, but evolutionary impacts. Such impacts had been a part of politics when Benjamin Franklin sent back seeds from Europe and Thomas Jefferson imported trees to Monticello, when George Washington set in motion his program of "internal improvements" to change the land and waters. They were present in the Westward Movement that has been aptly called the biological conquest of the continent, present in the park and forest programs of the early conservationists, present when the Congress passed a law making it the policy of the federal government to protect endangered species. The presence of such impacts has now become impossible to overlook, and we find ourselves in a new era of evolutionary governance.

This is a major change in the global political situation, a change in the nature of politics itself rather than the emergence of a new issue or set of issues. One of the most promising and most troublesome signs of this change is the phenomenon I have described as "creeping globalism"—promising in that it reveals the emergent outlines of a global polity, troublesome in that it threatens that explosive and fragile icon, national sovereignty. The growth of a new superstructure of global governance is a dramatic development in human history, but it still does not describe the entirety of the political transition now taking place.

The transition is producing, right in the uninformed midst of a public that believes itself to be reducing government, a quantitative increase in politics. There is simply more political interaction than there used to be, and more governance.

Politics, we have noted, requires certain basic ingredients: power, connection and uncertainty. There is no political interaction—no need for any laws, any structures of conflict resolution or allocation of value—where people have no contact, or where their interventions in nature do not affect other people. The Ohlone Indians on the shores of San Francisco Bay had no contact with the peoples on the other side of the Sierra and needed no political institutions in common. And until the issue of acid rain arose, somebody who drew fish from a lake in Norway had about as little interest in what the industries were up to over in England. Technological progress widens the circle of impact of individuals, companies, governments. For the impacts to become political they have to be known, of course; increasing information feeds the quantitative increase in politics. If the information were of the kind we once supposed scientific information to be—i.e., irrefutable certainty—there might be little or no increase in the kind of conflict and action we call politics. But everything is debatable, much is still unknown, much of what we know is in the form of probabilities and projections. Consequently debates about how to manage our ever-increasing power take place in the arena of values: the arena of politics.

Evolutionary Politics Now

I RECENTLY made a list, certainly not an all-inclusive one, of evolutionary concerns likely to be topics of public dialogue in the next couple of decades—and likely, I fear, to be present in the form of disasters large or small, problems out of control and tending to produce crisis-management responses. It includes:

- Adverse effects of deforestation, such as flooding and shortages of firewood.
- Overpopulation effects, including illegal migrations and overcrowded cities, and natural disasters—such as earthquakes and volcanic eruptions—which become massive human tragedies because of population density.
- Soil loss and desertification.

- Water shortages.
- Famines.
- Biological invaders (such as the Mediterranean Fruit Fly) that threaten agriculture or disrupt ecosystems.
- Water, soil, and air pollution.
- Pollution of oceans and diminution of fisheries.

I have not included in this list any such matters as global climate change, effects of nuclear war, or any of several other quite conceivable possibilities that do not, at the moment, appear to be absolutely certain future developments. All of the items on the above list are not really future scenarios at all. They are merely my unimaginative guess that things already happening will continue to happen. (My favorite futurist is the Kansas City pitcher Dan Quisenberry, who once remarked that the future is about like the present, only longer.)

As a supplement to the above list, here is another—of evolutionary matters less likely to be perceived as first-tier issues by the general public, but certain to be the subject of political dispute among special groups:

- Increasing species extinction.
- Management of species populations, where tradeoffs and conflicts of interest arise among different groups such as farmers, hunters, and preservationists.
- Loss of genetic resources, and control of genetic resources.
- Movement of plant and animal life around the world.
- Land use policy (one of the many areas in which major evolutionary consequences result from virtually unexamined public policies).

- Patenting and regulation of biotechnology and human reproductive technologies.
- Priorities in biotechnology.

These afford a glimpse of the territory, an idea of what some of the issues of evolutionary poltics are now and are likely to be in the future. Another way of approaching this subject is to consider the rather large number of *movements* that in one way or another deal with evolutionary and biopolitical causes. Among them are:

- The environmental movement, especially where it is concerned with global conditions and preservation of species or ecosystems.
- The animal rights movement.
- The population movement—Zero Population Growth, Planned Parenthood, and similar organizations.
- Anti-environmentalist or anti-population forces.
- Pro- and anti-abortion groups.
- Euthanasia and "right to die" movements.
- Anti-genetic technology efforts.
- Moves to regulate or outlaw various new reproductive technologies.
- New international initiatives, such as the agreement concerning free exchange of genetic material.
- Organizations advocating the teaching of creationism as an alternative to evolution.
- New spiritual and theological movements, such as those seeking to reconcile the evolution-creation dichotomy.
- Intellectual movements, such as the Association for Politics and the Life Sciences (a group of social scientists

interested in biopolitical research and theory) and the sociobiologists and their opponents.

I submit all these as evidence that evolutionary politics is not somewhere around the corner, but here. A general discovery of its presence will come about largely because we are forced to confront serious problems (most of them carry-overs from the days when people governed evolution without knowing it).

The Biological Revolution will be the other greatest single force in making us recognize the presence of evolutionary governance. We have managed so far to avoid knowing the extent of our interventions—but when we come to the point of conceiving human beings in laboratories, shipping the frozen embryos and semen of animals about the world, and planting forests of clones, it becomes impossible to continue hiding the truth from ourselves. This is the development I called "bioshock"—a change of unprecedented speed across a range of fields of human endeavor including those, such as agriculture and medicine, that most intimately connect to our daily lives and personal survival.

One commonly hears, in connection with the new biotechnologies, the breathless pronouncement that they bring us to the point of intervening in evolution itself. They do not: We had already reached that point when people learned how to make fires. What they really do is bring us to the point of *knowing* that we intervene in evolution. They mark the end of innocence—probably in a more spectacular and obvious way than the other processes of accelerated genetic change discussed in Chapter Three— and presage the beginning of a stage of human history in which, for the first time, it becomes part of the world-

view of the great majority of the human populatic
that the biological condition of the world is an evo
one, and (b) that human volition is a major force-
an ever-growing one—in determining the directic
change in the evolutionary process.

Some of the dangers that loom up before us a
contemplate this transition are external or ecological, h
to do with the health of the biosphere; others are int
human, having to do with stresses to individuals or soci

The dangers of the first type are relatively easy to c
and understand, for all the uncertainty of our data
despite our unwillingness to hear the news. We ca
deforestation and desertification. We can readily con
hend what people are telling us when they talk o
erosion, aquifer depletion, contamination by toxic cl
icals. We can read the reports from Worldwatch
Earthscan. We know these things are happening, an
have an increasing capacity to forecast what will r
from them. But the psychological dangers are hard
assess or predict. We have no way of knowing how p
will be affected by entry into an era of biological c
We have no Worldwatch Institute of the mind to te
how many people are threatened by change, how n
societies profoundly stressed beneath the surface.

What are the social and psychological dangers? Or
them, certainly, is the possibility that the Biological I
olution could be a largely two-tiered phenomenor
such a development educated elites will set priorities
biotechnology and agriculture, use new reproduc
technologies to bear healthy children, live long lives
tended through medicine and immunology, write r
lations for genetic screening and become terribly conce:
about endangered species and global ecology—while

[319]

majority of the people in the world struggle for daily survival in the crowded cities or try to produce food and firewood on minute plots of eroding land, and suffer from all the ills that the flesh (especially the flesh of poor people) has always been heir to. The danger I am trying to address here is not merely the problem of inequitable distribution of power and goods—which is serious enough—but something less familiar to political discourse. It has to do with the utter impossibility of achieving sound evolutionary governance by elites alone. However inequitable the distribution of power and information within human societies may be, the poorest human lords it over nature—can slaughter members of endangered species, relentlessly hack away forests in search of firewood, touch a match to an ecosystem in a piece of slash-and-burn agriculture. (Americans who need to be reminded of this might do well to carve into some Mount Rushmore the lad who, in 1900, did in the last wild passenger pigeon with a lucky shot from a bb gun.)

The realities of power in the biosphere are such that a successful transition into an era of responsible management of the planet can not be made merely by the educated and the fortunate, leaving everyone else to catch up later. If that happens (and to some extent it is happening now) we face the likelihood of a huge segment of the world's population displaced by various upheavals and movements from their cultures and environments, threatened and disaffected by the changes wrought by the Biological Revolution, and with no sense of connection to human society or the biosphere. Such a situation is a psychological tragedy that will in turn produce political tragedies and ecological ones.

The scenario that I have sketched out above is based on class and is only one way of looking at the possible social disruptions caused by rapidly increasing power and knowledge. If we dig a bit deeper into the human psyche, we can see yet another emerging polarization and another source of danger.

Notes on a Social Neurosis

IN *Civilization and its Discontents*, a classic study of the political animal's psychological predicament, Sigmund Freud worried that the future course of human progress might be "inextricably bound up with ... an increase of the sense of guilt, which will perhaps reach heights that the individual finds hard to tolerate."[3]

Freud was writing about the inward evolutionary struggle, the superego's attempt to subjugate sexual and aggressive drives in the service of civilized life. With the outcome of that evolutionary ordeal still much in doubt, we see now that it is the companion of yet another psychological dilemma. Each increase in human power and knowledge, each step in the subjugation of the external world that once held such danger and terror for primitive humanity, each reminder of the freedom of cultural choice that is now a part of our lives, brings an increase of the sense of reponsibility—which also may reach heights that the individual finds hard to tolerate.

The basic transition that the long march of human evolution represents—the transition from a pre-verbal existence among the other animals, the condition the political philosophers used to call the "state of nature," into civilization with its domesticated animals and its cultivated fields and its cities and its discontents—feels sometimes like victory, sometimes like defeat. The inner conflict is expressed in the persistent legends of a lost golden age, and in the myths of Genesis and Prometheus where knowledge is equated with sin and punishment. Evolution hurts; it is painful to the species over which we have claimed dominion, and it is painful to human beings— all the more so as we awaken to full comprehension of what we do and what has been done. There is, as C.G. Jung observed, no coming to consciousness without suffering.

We all know this at some level, yet shrink from the suffering. There are many manifestations of this avoidance abroad in our society, but the underlying denial of responsibility is the same. As we survey the field of contemporary evolutionary politics we can see two different extreme forms of avoidance: One is a flight into irresponsible dominance, a caricature of power; the other is a flight into irresponsible passivity, a caricature of innocence.

The first produces an exaltation of human control over nature, combined with a contempt toward efforts to encumber that control with legislation, regulation, or any morality beyond a few muddled Biblical maxims that justify exploitation as much as they moderate it. This evolutionary arrogance is manifested in many places, at many levels of society, in both secular and religious forms: the old-time Darwin, the old-time religion. In the Pacific Northwest there are lumberjacks riding about in pickups with guns hanging in the back windows and bumperstickers that say SIERRA CLUB KISS MY AXE. In corporate boardrooms, there are executives who, off the record and without bumperstickers, express similar views and act them out. In Washington, D.C. there are people who

kind of think humans can do whatever they want on—
or to—the oceans.

The second kind of flight generates a smug pseudo-
innocence, in which people displace onto others all responsibility for intervention while striving to convey the
impression that they, personally, have no more impact
upon the world than a butterfly and are profoundly in
tune with nature. It can be found among environmentalists—not so much among the movement's ecological
scientists or political activists, but frequently among those
who yearn to recapture the ecological wisdom of primitive
societies and search for non-anthropocentric modes of
relationship to nature. The aspiring "deep ecology"
movement is a good example of this, and of the sort of
cant it generates.[4]

People motivated by the dominance value system equate
reverence for life with reverence for human life; they will
go to any extreme to protect a human fetus, but are
indifferent toward the death or suffering of other organisms
or even the disappearance of entire species. They effortlessly
justify the cruelty of scientific experimentation with the
assumption that it saves human lives, and are infuriated
by efforts to halt or modify some construction project in
order to preserve an obscure species with a funny name.
(I have read many protests against endangered species
legislation which zero in on the fact that the species in
question have curious names like Furbish lousewort, as
if the names were ones the plants and animals had picked
out for themselves.) They revere (even if they misread)
the record of human intervention, and will countenance
no evidence that such intervention has produced anything
but progress. They freely express their aggressiveness toward nature—in hunting and fishing, for example—but

repress compassion for other life forms. A soft spot for a tame pet is tolerable, but the deeper and older sense of connection to all of life—which Edward Wilson calls "biophilia," an instinctive part of the human psyche—has no place in this consciousness.[5] Environmentalists are seen, from this point of view, as effete sentimentalists.

People who cling to the pose of innocence react against human life and are nervous about anything that might smack of anthropocentrism or speciesism. They admire anything that appears to be natural, but have trouble with the possiblity that any kind of intervention ever produces beneficial results. They are enchanted with bad news, ever on the lookout for another Prometheus to tie to the rocks. They freely (indeed ostentatiously) express compassion for other life forms but seem to be unaware of the hostility toward human life that comes out in their contempt for all their ancestors who have violated nature over the centuries, and in their willingness to belittle the work of environmentalists whose philosophy they find insufficiently pure. The deep ecology people dismiss virtually everything in the environmental movement—resource conservation, parklands and wilderness preservation, alternative technology, animal rights, and even the philosophy of Teilhard de Chardin—as "shallow ecology."[6] This is a mode of discourse long favored by intellectuals on the make; it is strongly reminiscent of the good old days when Marxists of varying shades verbally pummelled one another in the drawing rooms of London over who possessed the purer strain of revolutionary thought, and hearkens back to yet earlier times when the question was salvation and the name of the game was Holier Than Thou. Yet it has a distinctly late-twentieth-century content, and strikingly illustrates one strategy for escaping from the anguish of the human condition, one attempt to opt out of the collective wrong-doing of the species. And it reflects a profound bitterness and alienation; behind the claim to a superior form of biophilia lurks old-fashioned misanthropy.

Both extreme forms of our common social neurosis reflect a deep-seated pain, a condition of knowing (even if not admitting) that the human evolutionary struggle has been attended by enormous suffering and destruction—suffering of other forms of life, of the Earth, and of human beings as well. The psychological conflict involved in human intervention in nature is at least as stressful as that involved in the other evolutionary struggle, the one Freud and the psychoanalysts deal with, between the instinctual and the symbolic sides of the human psyche. The extremes of reaction, the fantasies of control and the fantasies of innocence, only mark the boundaries of something that encompasses us all: a persistent unwillingness to come to terms with the totality of the human condition. This condition is one of great accomplishment and promise, and also of something very like original sin.

It is an old problem, in a way: A century ago Lord Acton observed that power tends to corrupt and absolute power corrupts absolutely. He was quite right, but so is Edgar Z. Friedenberg's more recent response:"All weakness tends to corrupt, and impotence corrupts absolutely."[7]

Rollo May has written of a recurrent pattern of pseudo-innocence, common to the human race but particularly evident in American life, where it takes the form of a conscious denial of power:

The denial of our desires for power, when it occurs in the endeavor to cover up an actually high degree of power, sets up an inner contradiction: power does not allay our *feelings of powerlessness*. It does not lead to the sense of responsibility that actual power ought to entail. We cannot develop responsibility for what we don't *admit* we have. We cannot act upon our power directly, for we always carry an element of guilt at having it. If we were to admit it, we would have to confront our guilt.[8]

This applies, certainly, to the meatless-and-guiltless form of pseudo-innocence, which is sustainable only by repressing awareness of the enormous outlays of power that are part of the historical past and the daily existence of *every* person in Western civilization. But as you go more deeply into the thinking—and especially the writing—of those on the other side who unapolegetically praise human power in nature, it turns out that there is a pseudo-innocence there also: All uses of power are seen as benign adjustments, never as rapacious or destructive acts. "Internal improvements" has been the durable American euphemism for anything done to the continent. The deliberate extinction of species is never acknowledged, and if the subject arises the human act is likened to an event of Darwinian inevitability, devoid of human intention. Impacts are edged away from, responsibility diluted in reassuring words. Those laboratory animals don't feel anything, those animals on the farm have plenty to eat. It is something like the slaveholder's confidence that the darkies were happy.

It is an old game, but it takes on a new dimension in relation to our behavior as citizens of the biosphere. There is guilt involved, certainly, in accepting the truth that we are all products of countless past acts of violence toward the planet and its life—and not only in the past, but in the web of life that we are connected to today. But there is also responsibility, the burden of being constantly re-minded of our connections to one another and to the rest of life. It is a responsibility we greatly want to resist, and that resistance will be a stubborn part of the evolutionary politics that is rapidly becoming the context of all our lives.

The Struggle of Power and Innocence

I HAVE BEEN deliberately describing the more extreme forms of response to the situation, because the situation will quite likely be one to provoke extreme responses. We should expect not only strong feelings and intense political conflict, but also irrationality and violence.

Some of the heat will come from people who unques-tioningly accept human dominance in nature. When people of that persuasion find their activities hampered by en-vironmental restrictions, for example, their reaction can be one of extreme anger. Anyone who doubts my word on this point is invited to chat with a farmer who has to deal with pesticide regulations or a developer blocked from building on his land. We have already seen a strong anti-environmentalist movement during the Reagan years, strong enough to capture such citadels of power as the Environmental Protection Administration and undermine much of its work. The volume of environmental regulation will continue to increase for many years to come, and this may be, to put it mildly, disappointing to people who have been led to expect that there will be less. There may well continue to be a move toward deregulation in some areas, but the pace of human impacts will make environmental regulation a growth industry of governance;

[327]

many people are not going to like that at all, and we will hear from them.

On another front, we have already seen the rise of a large and powerful and devoted anti-abortion movement, attended by occasional outbreaks of violence such as bombings of abortion clinics. More of this is inevitable. The development of new abortifacient and contraceptive technologies and the wider reliance by many people on embryo transplant and related reproductive methods will complicate this picture but in no way reduce the intensity of feelings about it. The conflict over population and birth control is now expanding in scale, and promises to become a huge controversy, with global networks of activists on both sides fighting for the hearts and minds—not to mention the reproductive organs—of people around the world.

Look for a similar global polarization over endangered species and the protection/management/use of them. We are moving toward a time when every ecosystem in the world will be subject to management by some government (one could make a good case that we are there already) and when the survival of every species, endangered or not, will be affected by public policy. The recognition that such a highly managed state of nature exists is likely to disturb the kinds of people who resent obstacles to human use and development of land; and also will be less than satisfactory to many environmentalists who would rather see plants and animals allowed to live in pure wilderness conditions, unencumbered by any human meddling. It will provoke conflict between groups, and there are many ways that it can produce violence and/or require harsh law-enforcement measures—against poachers, for example.

It may be harder to foresee disturbances in the political system caused by people on the innocence side of the spectrum, who disclaim a desire for power in nature— but I think its explosive potential is vastly underrated. When you do not consider yourself to be personally guilty of exerting power over nature it is an easy step to view others as very guilty indeed, and to be prepared to take extreme action to halt their crimes. This is the moral logic that enables people to bomb abortion clinics in the name of reverence for life, and it can equally well be used to justify extreme action in the cause of, say, animal rights or global ecology.

Animal rights activism teeters frequently on the edge of violence and, although most of the movement's leaders profess a Gandhian orientation, there are others—such as Hans Ruesch, author of *Slaughter of the Innocent*, who believes that violent assault on scientists who use animals in research is morally justifiable.[9] Another kind of militant environmentalism has become increasingly visible. Its textbook is Edward Abbey's *The Monkey Wrench Gang*, a story about a group of eco-guerrillas who went from destroying billboards to trying to blow up a dam. It has recently surfaced in the form of a group called Earth First! which defines itself as "the conscience of the environmental movement." Its founder has written a book that includes suggestions for "fun and easy" ways to play the game of "eco-sabotage."[10]

I have a hard time with such political rhetoric. It is true that much of what the Earth Firsters advocate is merely the destruction of other forms of destruction, and I have yet to see a billboard that would not look better lying down than standing up. But I am troubled, as I hear the eco-guerrilla talk, by the unacknowledged arrogance it expresses, the certainty of rightness. I am troubled also, as I observe the progress of the crusade against biotechnology, by the violence—not yet a violence of action, but a violence of rhetoric, a desire to dramatize and simplify issues and crank up the moral intensity of controversy so that it becomes, instead of a dialogue between people with different opinions, an Armaggedon between the forces of good and the forces of evil. I read Jeremy Rifkin's prose in which he announces that what the world needs is more empathy, and then I note his tendency to deal with people he disagrees with as if they were evil incarnate.[11] That kind of a stance toward the world—a hard core of misanthrophy wrapped in professions of moral superiority—is one that has historically wrought great mischief in times of political upheaval.

These various expressions of power and innocence reflect the basic political polarization of the Biological Revolution. The basic polarization that emerged from the Industrial Revolution was free enterprise v. collectivism, with a strong class base to conflict. The new polarization is rooted in the psyche—in the ancient struggle to come to terms with human power in nature—and it takes the form of conflict in the political arena between those who hold human dominance to be either unassailably rational or God-ordained, and those who are sickened by the wrongness of much of what humans have done in the biosphere. It is an outward conflict which reflects something that lives within every one of us. It may well take the form of principled dialogue and bring us all to a new understanding, and it may also be marred with destructive battle as people hammer at each other about half-truths. It is a kind of conflict that provides a rich breeding-ground for demagogues, a feast of justification for drastic action.

There is, unfortunately, no basis in human history for confidence that the opening of a new season of ethical conflict in politics will make politics itself more ethical. We have done some of our ugliest work around high causes.

As new polarizations emerge they do not replace old ones, but interpenetrate them and complicate the world political picture. The Industrial Revolution is still rolling along its endlessly innovative path, and the perennial clash between collectivism and free enterprise now appears in new contexts: conflicts over the control of genetic resources, over biotechnology, over the minerals in the oceans. In most of these the adversarial lineup is not Western allies versus Communist bloc, but rather developed nations vs. Third World, have vs. have-not. In place of the bipolar world of the Cold War we have a multipolar one. Some alignments are defined in the familiar terms of class and national interest. Others express the different ways that people react to the psychological stresses of the Biological Revolution. To further complicate the matter, the Information Revolution makes it possible for new networks and coalitions to emerge rapidly, so that polarizations about major issues—such as population—quickly move into a global scale. Such polarizations may be understandable in some geographic context—East-West, North-South—or they may be quite lacking in a sense of place, mobile as a multinational corporation or a popular song.

There are many sources of conflict. The biosphere is in serious trouble: It is rapidly losing much of its genetic resources, its forests and soil and air and water are contaminated, its human population is still increasing at an unprecedented pace. The gap is growing between the human haves and the human have-nots, and—less noticed—

between the human race and the rest of the world as human power in nature increases. The world is biologically, culturally, politically and economically unstable; technological change challenges old value systems, creates new contexts and new problems, and places still more power in the keeping of organizations and individuals.

A forbidding picture. The dangers are apparent enough. The opportunities may be harder to see from this point of view, but the very conditions which unsettle our lives have the promise of being wrought into efforts of high purpose and great benefit. The opportunities, like the dangers, need to be considered on a new scale.

The Largest Undertaking of All Time: A Modest Proposal

THE EARTH'S health and productivity is declining at an alarming rate: spreading desertification in many areas, massive soil erosion, dismal expanses of newly-leveled tropical forests, contamination of air and ground and water. No country in the world is untouched by it, and some countries (including at least two neighbors of the United States, Haiti and El Salvador) are close to ecological collapse. The immense inertial force of ecological destruction has not noticeably slackened in the environmental decades, and many who study it have been driven to the bleak conclusion that it will roll on well into the next century.

Yet, even while the damage continues, you can find in many parts of the world a surprising amount of movement in the opposite direction: evidence that it is not necessary to wait for the end of the population wave or the coming of Ecotopia to begin a new chapter in the history of human creation of artificial ecosystems. It is possible to talk seriously about renewing the Earth. Much renewal

[332]

work has been done and is being done now, although mostly at a slow pace and a local scale.

One of the earliest regional restoration projects in the United States dates from the late 1930s, the time just after the great dust storms in the southwestern plains. The federal government set in motion a program aimed at developing new farming techniques that would hold the ground, and persuading farmers to use them. The program also reseeded thousands of acres with grass and planted thousands of trees as windbreaks and watershed stabilizers.

Today ecosystem restoration has become a widespread activity in the United States, part movement and part scientific discipline. It has its own journal, *Restoration and Management Notes*, and some of its successes were chronicled in a 1985 book, *Restoring the Earth*[12] Among the heroes of the movement are the master marsh builder of Chesapeake Bay, Ed Garbish, whose work in transforming wasted shorelines into healthy wetland ecosystems in the midst of a heavily traveled waterway shows that environmental reconstruction can coexist with conventional economic uses.

The essence of a restoration project is not necessarily duplication of an ecosystem that once existed, (although many impressive efforts of that sort can be found) but the deliberate creation of artificial ecosystems that have a higher degree of complexity and stability than the ecosystems human beings have generally designed in the past.

Such projects are underway in many places. Consider the Yijinholo region of Mongolia, site of the tomb of Genghis Khan, half a world away from the American dust bowl. Yijinholo was once a place of forest and green pasture, but over centuries of the kind of misuse that is common on every continent—overfarming by growing

[333]

populations, ploughing of grassland, deforestation, unrestrained grazing of cattle and sheep—it became a near-wasteland. Trees disappeared, hundreds of square miles of pasture became shifting sand dunes. Crop production declined, and fierce sandstorms killed thousands of cattle. Then, in 1974, the local population and the government began a program of restoration. They fenced in grazing areas, restricted the size of herds, planted trees and grass on the sand dunes, slowly and painstakingly reclaimed the land. Within ten years forest cover had spread over nearly a quarter of the region, grain yields had increased, and flocks were no longer dying off in sandstorms.[13]

Consider a project down on the eastern coast of Costa Rica, started by a couple of North American ecological entrepreneurs. The keystone of it is a boat called the "ocean pickup," a sail-powered commercial vessel, fast and seaworthy but simple in design. A prototype has performed impressively in the fisheries of South and Central America. Catching fish is only a part of the payoff, however. The enterprise is a piece of integrated development—with small local shipbuilding factories to construct more ocean pickups, and local forests growing trees to build them. The goals: to revive a depressed fishing industry in an area where (as in much of the Third World) artisan-fishermen have become dependent on foreign machinery, foreign parts, and foreign petroleum; to create a new local shipbuilding industry; and to do some commercial re-forestation in a country that is rapidly using up its trees.[14]

Note that the work is both economic development and ecosystem restoration. Note, too, that it draws on a body of scientific research and involves planting of imported fast-growing trees selected because of their usefulness for this particular purpose. It is an intentional design of an

economy/ecosystem, in some ways technologically sophisticated and linking the local fishermen to the most
advanced developments in one area of global culture (the
ocean pickup's designer is a New England naval architect
who learned his craft building racing boats), and in some
ways quite simple and meant to *dis*engage the local fishing
industry from the global petroleum economy.

Even in Brazil, a country in the process of bringing off
one of the largest accomplishments in ecological *mis*-
management the world has yet seen—the destruction of
the Amazon forest, itself an impressive demonstration of
how much ecological change can be achieved in a short
time—there are intriguing signs of movement in another
direction. If you fly over that ravaged land you see pieces
of tropical forest standing undisturbed. They are not precisely sights of beauty, those islands amid the waste, but
they represent a significant effort: The Brazilian environmental agency, SEMA, has established a network of environmental stations surrounded by forest, ranging in size
from one hectare (2.47 acres) to 1800 hectares (3.8 square
miles). By law, 90 percent of this land is to be preserved
intact as a living "genetic bank," and 10 percent is to be
used for research on burning, ecological succession, and
other aspects of ecosystem management. One of the ob-
jectives is simply to find out what is the real size of an
ecosystem in that region, how small an area can be preserved
and still exist when surrounded by cleared land.[15]

There is no region for which there are not restoration
methods to build more complex and stable ecosystems,
increase organic productivity, and reduce pollution. Some
of the methods are ancient, and some are new approaches
emerging along with the rest of the Biological Revolution.
There are ways to create living gene banks, to clean up

lakes and rivers, to develop agricultural systems that do not erode soil and pollute water—even ways to build ecological cities. Although urban restoration lags behind other renewal technologies in practice, many innovations can be found: landscaped rooftops, warehouses converted to food gardens, fish growing in fiberglass containers.[16] In *Restoring the Earth*, the author describes an imaginary city whose airport is "paved" with a genetically engineered plant; it provides a tough, smooth and impermeable ground cover, and also, through photosynthesis, makes a contribution to the atmosphere. A touch fanciful, but not too far beyond the possible.

Sooner or later, restoration work will become a universal global activity, with a growing body of knowledge, worldwide networks of information exchange, and the participation of great numbers of people. It is well within our reach to make it that immediately, because the same change in political scale that causes us such distress also enables us to conceive and commence very large undertakings quickly. It is quite possible for a project of global restoration to emerge into the world culture before the end of the century; possible for a message to go out through the mass media about the first human project, a common effort to repair the foundation of all our lives.

I am quite serious in describing this as a modest proposal. It will be, of course, the largest undertaking that the human race has ever engaged in, unless one counts the transformation of the planet that we have already achieved, over a period of thirty thousand years or so: I mean the burst of activity in an instant of evolutionary time that moved rice from its place of origin in Asia to fields around the world, eliminated thousands of species of plant and animal life, remodeled the faces of continents, changed

[336]

the patterns of waterways, chased the bison from the plains of North America, planted European grasses on the valley floors of California—and brought to my immediate neighborhood such diverse life forms as Europeans, Asians, Africans, Latin Americans, eucalyptus trees, the tomato plants in my garden and the calico cat that sleeps in my greenhouse window. We have made the world over once and it is time to make it over again, this time in decades, with better understanding of how ecosystems work and with global information transfer.

There are more precedents than we might at first expect for large-scale social undertakings, with or without an ecological dimension. The rebuilding of the North American continent was one such; the crash conversion of the U.S. peacetime economy into a war machine in the months after Pearl Harbor is another. The latter is a good case history of the creation not only of a new industrial system but a new culture, steeped in the values and beliefs of the war effort, inspired by the Hollywood mythmakers. Yet another precedent worthy of our attention is the Marshall Plan, one of the more notable successes of American foreign policy, which was designed to restore the war-ravaged economic and industrial base of Europe. The United States could easily set in motion an ecological Marshall Plan or several of them—one for Africa, for example, another for Central America—as a unilateral step in the direction of the larger undertaking which must involve all nations, the entire community of organizations and non-organizations which is the de facto global polis.

As there are many small projects already doing the work of Earth renewal, so are there larger conceptualizations that seek to tie such efforts together: the United Nations Environmental Programme is one, the tropical forests restoration project that has been launched by a coalition of environmental groups is another. The new network of intergovernmental and nongovernmental organizations provides a framework for coordinating activities and sharing information, and scientific networks such as the one envisioned for the International Geosphere-Biosphere Program provide a necessary information base. The work will be, to an unprecedented extent, a work of information exchange and technology transfer. It will also call for adopting a model of "economic development" that does not require destruction of the living infrastructure in the search for short-term payoffs.

In that effort we will have an opportunity to look at projects of different kinds and sizes, from large ones of the sort that the modern era is famous (or infamous) for, to small ones based on the ethic of bioregionalism and appropriate technology. I suspect we will find in practice that there are many ways to combine the two—that it will turn out to be possible to do small-is-beautiful restoration work on a large scale.

We may also find it possible to discover some common ground beneath the ideological gap now widening between the culture of dominance and the culture of innocence. Just as there is a common source for the extreme positions— an inability to come to terms with human responsibility in nature—so is there a common source for all the things— good and bad, caring and rapacious—that people do to the Earth. Call it creativity, the universal human urge to participate in an act of creation, to do something more with the Earth than merely inhabit it. Like other deep human drives (see sex) it can take many forms, from sublime to obscene. It motivates developers and farmers and landscape architects and the ordinary householder placing bulbs in the soil. Environmental purists rail at it and often with good reason, but then I read that the founder of Earth First! wants to reintroduce grizzly bears into the Marble Mountains of California. Another improvement project. It is true that this one is in the service of recreating something like the ecosystem of 200 years back, but to do it in the late years of the twentieth century requires importing bears, looking over their shoulders as they breed and rear their young, keeping track of their movements, protecting them from humans and protecting humans from them. Not only an improvement project, but a piece of evolutionary governance, requiring the support of state and federal agencies and public funds.

Consider, as one final example of a piece of Earth renewal, a prairie in Illinois. Illinois calls itself the Prairie State, but examples of true prairie ecosystems are hard to find there. The best example is the one on the property of the Fermi National Accelerator Laboratory—occupying 650 acres in the center of the proton accelerator ring. It is very similar to what the original prairies looked like, with waving grasses six feet tall, blossoming wildflowers, ground squirrels and sandhill cranes and trumpeter swans. The prairie was built there. It was built through the labor of prairie restoration experts who plowed and disked the ground to get rid of weeds and planted seeds with a Nesbit drill, and also through the labor of over a hundred volunteers who helped with the work of harvesting seeds of native prairie plants, and sometimes putting them in the ground by hand.[17] You do not get a prairie in Illinois today by fencing off a piece of land and waiting for the grass to grow back. If you do that you get an interesting collection of weeds from all over the world. The prairie is there because many people passionately wanted to build it.

That creative drive, the urge to dig and plant and mold the Earth, is the source of all our problems and it may well be the source of our solutions, the energy that can be tapped for a work of a size and scale and beauty beyond anything we have yet attempted.

I do not mean that in this effort all our differences will disappear. The decades ahead will be difficult ones, whatever we undertake. But it is possible that there is much to be gained in coming finally to face the Earth and our profoundly different ideas about what to do with it. That very conflict can be in itself productive. It is not the path which is our difficulty, Kierkegaard said: rather, it is our difficulty which is the path. And perhaps the dangers are the opportunity.

The work of restoration offers a place to discover some common ground—if we cannot find it in the Earth we will never find it anywhere—and a way to make clearer and more accessible the larger challenge that we will face in the time ahead, of creating a human society commensurate to our power in the world. It will bring into common currency some understanding of the possibilities of the Biological Revolution and the workings of ecosystems, and it will bring agendas for future global development— competing visions of what the Earth may become—into the common political dialogue.

I am trying to give an image here not of a completed product, but rather of a kind of process, at once political and ecological, that it is within the human grasp to begin. In such a process many things will be tried, there will be failures and successes of all kinds, and much will be learned.

Many exciting events are unfolding now, and many signs of hope blossoming in the troubled biosphere. We are all witnesses at the breech birth of a global society; we are in the midst of a profound scientific/technological revolution that promises great new advances in medicine and agriculture and industry. There is good reason to believe that within the forty-year crisis period ahead— within it, not after it—we can eliminate many major diseases; bring food production and distribution to the point of ending the malnutrition which is now rampant; vastly reduce the number of children born with severe birth defects; make birth control materials and information available to everyone; create methods of economic development that will reverse the slide into unemployment and homelessness which is now the lot of so many millions; and, for the first time in human history, begin an upward curve in the quality of life for the other sentient beings with which we share the planet. Opportunities, indeed.

Life and Governance in the Postmodern World

ALTHOUGH the biopolitical events that are taking place in the world are monumentally complex and include developments moving in precisely opposite directions—ecosystem restoration concurrent with ecosystem destruction, for example—it is possible to pick out certain overriding themes that define the conditions of life and governance in our time.

One of these is the change of scale. The globalizing part of that change is perhaps the easiest to see and understand. The "placeless" communities created by the Information Revolution are a bit harder to grasp. The change of time scale—in our time—may be the hardest of all.

We can see the curve arc upward through many kinds of data—species extinction, human population growth, technological innovation, international organizations—but may not immediately comprehend that it is presenting us with situations to which we must respond, whether personally or collectively, with speed and flexibility. The Biological Revolution will unfold much more rapidly than the Industrial Revolution did—thanks in large part to the Information Revolution which is the bridge between the two.

A second overriding trend is the one that I described in this chapter as an escalation of intentionality: more things determined by conscious human choice. It comes with an increase in the *quantity* of political interactions with a greater volume of interconnections, information, and uncertainty. It leads to an increasing centrality of moral, ethical and religious dialogue in the political arena. The same process alters the nature of personal life and in fact blurs the distinction between the personal and political as the most private actions—like conceiving and dying—become charged with new choices and new ideological conflicts.

The third major trend is the increasing primacy of learning. It is so central to evolutionary governance that education is one of the first things we must address as a matter of public policy, that learning becomes a central prop of a biopolitical culture, and that a program of Earth restoration is to be seen as a global learning project. We need overarching concepts that help us make sense of our world, that structure our thinking about what is happening and what is to be done; an idea of ongoing learning is fundamental to that.

All these comments point toward our being in new, unfamiliar, and quite different political territory. Stephen Toulmin, to whom I am indebted for the use of the term "postmodern," says that we no longer live in the modern world, but rather in a "postmodern world"—the world, as he puts it, "that has not yet discovered how to define itself in terms of what it is, but only in terms of what it has *just-now ceased to be.*"[18]

I am not particularly enchanted with the idea, favored by many futurists, that the transition into the postmodern world is best explained as a paradigm shift. Thomas Kuhn's description of what happens in scientific revolutions—that one view of reality reigns for a time while anomalies accumulate, then a new explanatory model arises and displaces the old one—has been extended by several writers into a scheme of cultural evolution. Usually it is posited that we are moving into a post-Cartesian and post-Newtonian world-view, much more holistic and systemic— and, in most versions, with a new ecological value system.[19]

There is no doubt that it is becoming much more necessary to view the Earth as a whole system—indeed, the biological interconnections are increasing at a much greater rate than the new-paradigm theorists suspect—but our present encounter with that reality is not the same thing as the sweeping transformation of global consciousness described in the new-paradigm literature.

The notion of paradigm shift once seemed to me a persuasive explanation of how values and beliefs change in societies; but after living with the matter for a decade or so I have come to believe that as a model of large-scale social change it is oversimplified and dangerously prone to wishful thinking. It promises a lot of rose gardens.

[343]

I am not surprised that Kuhn himself did not recommend its use outside the history of science.

One of the shortcomings is that people who favor it tend to believe that they are in possession of the new paradigm, and that human progress is measurable in terms of conversion of other people to their value system. (I have met many conservatives and not a few outright reactionaries, but I have yet to meet anybody who professed to hold an old paradigm.) The more serious problem is that it is essentially a model of clear transition: a revolution in thought followed by a new order which brings a period of consolidation. In Kuhn's description the new paradigm takes over and becomes accepted framework of thought for a new establishment. The paradigm is dead, long live the paradigm.

I would be delighted to see humanity make some such unmuddied leap from one ethos to the next, but it appears to me that the best model we have available for what is now happening is not Kuhn's description of paradigm shifts in the sciences but rather the familiar exponential curve. The phenomenon of increasing rates of change is evident in so many aspects of contemporary life that it requires no great act of faith to view it as likely to continue through the near-term future. The exponential growth of technological innovation is a particularly well-documented and pervasive example. In view of this, I think we would do well to consider that we are not so much on the brink of a paradigm shift as somewhere on the middle slopes of a very steep social learning curve—and that *all* people will be required to take in new information, modify values and beliefs, and meanwhile (as we noted in the discussion of culture) modify meta-ideas *about* information, values, and beliefs. We learn to live on the curve.

[344]

The curve becomes a much more interesting environment to inhabit when we understand that the process is not only one of taking in data, but of giving meaning and purpose to life. When the philosophers speak of intentionality they do not merely mean action taken deliberately instead of inadvertently, choices consciously made, but also life lived in a larger context of meaning. Whatever we may bring into the world in the way of ethic, ideology or ecological mystique will have to rest upon comprehension of the human/global condition. Ultimately we will require a world-view which is both religious and evolutionary; more immediately and fundamentally, we require a shared sense of participation in what I have described as the human econiche.

The econiche of any plant or animal, its biological job description, is defined in terms of its relationship to other plants and animals. An ecosystem is an arrangement of econiches, in much the same way that an organization is an arrangement of roles; sometimes a species will enter an ecosystem, displace an incumbent from its position, and the ecosystem's life goes on more or less as before. The uniqueness of the human species lies in having developed the capability to relate to the system as a whole—and consequently to all life forms and to all ecosystems. And the chief difference between the world of today and the world of a few thousand years ago is that it now possesses such a species. This is a very great difference indeed, one which transforms the biosphere.

The human species is, by virtue of its econiche, in a different category from all other forms of life—yet intimately bound to all other life forms. Peter A. Corning, in one of the more interesting of the many recent attempts to create a post-Darwinian concept of evolution, theorizes that the overall direction of evolutionary progress is guided neither by lonely selfishness as in the classical "survival of the fittest" model, nor by the Grand Plan of a single external intelligence, but by synergy—that is, by interaction and interdependence, including many kinds of deliberate co-operation among different life forms.[20] If this is so, then humanity's rise is to be understood in terms of its ability to interact creatively with other living things, and its future success will rest on its ability to improvise entirely new ways to do this. This improvisation will be essentially a political process; in much the same way that the species moved out of barbarism into civilization by creating government and laws, it will move into evolutionary responsibility by creating new principles, policies, ideologies and institutions.

This puts the human species in a very central place in the biosphere. The perspective that I offer here is strongly and frankly anthropocentric. Yet I do not see any reason to believe that the human species was destined for this role; other species have their own forms of culture and symbolic communication and might quite likely have advanced to the pan-interactional econiche if *Homo sapiens* had not arrived there first. Nor do I see any evidence to persuade me that the human species is descended from some supernatural or extraterrestrial life form, as is sometimes speculated.[21] If we reject such an exotic explanation, we are left with a homelier—but ultimately far more mysterious—account: that Earth itself brought forth human intelligence and that all the biopolitical events of our time, from the Endangered Species Act to test tube babies, are parts of nature and parts of the biosphere's troubled metamorphosis.

[346]

We are still within nature. But we are no longer within the nature our distant ancestors knew, where life was driven solely by instinct, the years came and went unchangingly, and it was unthinkable that the global environment could be altered by human action. We have come out of that garden into a different kind of existence, into a world created not only by the hand of God but also by the actions of countless other people, past and present. And exile from the garden turns out to be not a single event but an ongoing process: Every day, the course of events carries us farther out into the world in which we know, and act, and know we act. Every day is Genesis.

We can choose to know many different things, and we can choose to act in many different ways. But we cannot choose not to know, or not to act. It is a painful experience to come to consciousness of this kind of a world, but we cannot long delay doing so. All the actions are already in progress, and we most need a sense of meaning that will give them structure and enable us to proceed into a world in which governance is understood as something that takes place not just within the human species but in the entire biosphere, with the human species playing a different role from other species. We cannot wait too long to enter fully into this new and unfamiliar terrain, to take on the huge learning task that it presents. We have everything to lose, and a world to build.

[Epilogue]

Participatory Evolution:
Thoughts for the Activist,
Acts for the Thinker

MY PRIMARY purpose has been to sketch a general outline of the political territory we are now entering, not to prescribe a specific set of public policies for governments or a how-to guide for the aspiring biopolitical activist. Yet I understand the feelings of those who, having seen the terrain, want to ask the question that Lenin asked when he surveyed post-revolutionary Russia and contemplated the possibilities: What is to be done?

I hope that I have provided at least a few partial answers to that question. We have seen many things that are either (a) urgently in need of doing or (b) already being done and urgently in need of recognition that we are doing them. But those are only fragments at best and for those who would pursue the search further I would like to look at the territory again from a slightly different perspective.

First, let us consider the various problems and issues and movements discussed in the foregoing chapter as a set of *projects*—evolutionary/political undertakings that have already been begun. The list includes:

- The Earth restoration project.
- The eugenics project: attempts to guide human evolution through genetic screening, birth control, reproductive technologies, directed breeding programs (i.e., sperm banks with selected donors), and extraordinary medical measures to maintain the lives of premature and defective newborn children.
- The population project: the attempt to place a limit on the growth of human numbers by reducing birth rates.
- The genetic resources project: the attempt to maintain a store of genetic information—whether by ecosystem preservation, gene banking or any other method. This includes protecting species from extinction and protecting specific populations or individuals. It overlaps to some extent 'with:
- The animal rights project: the attempt to promulgate throughout human societies (and governments) a general idea of the rights of animals and other living things, and to protect species from extinction without concern for their immediate usefulness to humans.
- The genetic technology project: attempts to create new forms of life, speed up mutation and the development of new species, and produce new vaccines and therapeutic methods.

This is not an exhaustive list of the evolutionary adventures upon which people are embarked, but it covers the main lines of current activity. Each cries out for greater understanding and a deeper involvement of private citizens and public officials—not only because there is work such as genetic resource conservation that needs support, but also because some of the projects are lurching along with little visible sense of direction. This is particularly true of eugenics, where the lack of public dialogue about what might be done is perpetuated by the widespread belief that eugenics itself is a curiosity of past history. Several of the projects that I have enumerated could be subsumed under the larger project of biosphere management, which includes such activities as maintaining populations of wild animals and dealing with human impacts on the oceans and the atmosphere. And over and above such causes is the larger adventure, the master project of creating a structure of institutions and culture than can serve as the vessel for such acts and agendas. Certainly there is much to be done, but there is more to it than that:

What we are encountering now is not only the emergence of some new issues, but an alteration in the nature of politics: a change in *scale*, a change in *content*, and a change in *modes* of political action. This is something the political activist needs to understand, and the effort to understand it restores the connection between political thought and action—a connection that has been eroding in the modern world where people have become increasingly eager to get busy and suspicious of intellectualizing. Unless we strive continuously to comprehend the distinct character of the postmodern world—to think as clearly as we can— our actions are in danger of being misguided or counterproductive, and those of us who really aren't interested in political action will be rudely surprised to find that we are being acted upon.

As a result of the change in scale of political time and space, the major developments of history become more immediate and inclusive. Things move quickly, and nobody remains untouched for long.

The master projects of earlier civilizations were more localized geographically and slower to unfold. The philosophers of Athens were trying to make discoveries for the whole human race, but people a few hundred miles away knew little of their aspirations. The medieval enterprise of building a Christian polis on Earth was similarly cosmic in conception, but it was chiefly a European activity. While crusaders and kings marched across the land, while thinkers plumbed the depths of reality, while grandiose projects arose and fell, much of humanity stood apart and watched. Some people were touched directly by such doings, more were touched indirectly, and many never knew of them at all.

But throughout the modern era the distance between people, states, cultures and ecosystems has been shrinking. Amid the confusions and conflicts a transition has been taking place—the emergence of a global society. And in the closing years of the twentieth century we are entering a new era, a postmodern era in which that transition is, for all practical purposes, complete. I don't mean that we have achieved a stable situation—far from it—but rather that we have progressed into another chapter of human history, in which the entire biosphere is a single political system.

We were ushered into the postmodern era by the atomic bomb, that anomalous weapon created to be an instrument of national security but now demonstrating so vividly the limitations of the nation-state. The vision of global atomic war held up a mirror to the human race in which the species stood revealed to itself—for the first time—as capable of doing something that would affect the whole world immediately, with nobody left out. Some see the nuclear threat as in a class by itself and expect that if it were removed we would again have the luxury of living in a more private and leisurely kind of world. But the bomb is merely the most spectacular of many ways that we are capable of destroying the Earth; and, once we have attained the capacity to destroy the Earth, we have perforce taken on the obligation to maintain it. That maintenance—whether achieved simply by not blowing the world up or by not destroying its ozone layer, or achieved in more positive and creative ways by restoring its beauty and health and productivy—becomes one of the central political activities of our time. There is no way of reversing the sequence of historical developments that have made the biosphere an object of political concern.

Globalism and exponential change are the framework within which the political animal must now go about its business. Within that framework, we have new *issues*—matters like genetic resources and animal rights and all the promises and perils of the Biological Revolution—that present themselves to us as matters to be dealt with by state and local and national governments, and also by the various international bodies that have emerged as parts of the global system of governance. We will see new issues, and we will also see the Biological Revolution sometimes transforming the economic and class-based concerns of the past. For example, a biotechnological process for relatively cheap artificial production of sugar has already had an impact on the economies of some sugar-producing countries. Let us imagine what might happen if—as is entirely possible—sugar cane becomes no longer worth growing. This would be initially disastrous, in reducing a source of foreign exchange and employment in many Third World countries, but it would also make vast amounts of land available for food production or reforestation. The problem of allocating priorities in biotechnology will turn out to be far more politically complex than merely directing energy toward tropical diseases and Third World agriculture; it will lead along many paths to large-scale ecological management.

Scale itself—especially where new supranational organizations might be called for—becomes one of the issues. As the Biological Revolution unfolds, the issues it presents will be very hard to contain within our present arrangement of levels of government. We have always had jurisdictional disputes and ideological debate about what ought properly to be done at what level, but we haven't seen anything yet.

Consider the eugenics project: In California (as in several other states and several other countries) we now have sperm banks. We even have left-wing sperm banks and right-wing sperm banks. The Feminist Women's Health Center in Oakland accepts donations from anonymous males including homoxesuals and serves childless married couples, unmarried women and lesbians; its effect is to make biological parenthood available to many people living nontraditional lifestyles. The Repository for Germinal Choice in Escondido seeks donations from Nobel Prize winners and serves women who are interested in giving birth to intellectually superior children. Its agenda is admittedly elitist—and explicitly eugenic. It is a small, local, and duly licensed private business, observing all the appropriate regulations, and its business activity is directed human evolution. Are the local and state regulations sufficient to deal with the public interest questions raised by such an enterprise, or should there be some prevailing national policy concerning directed human evolution? On the other hand, should these decisions be regarded as entirely within the province of individual right? Conceiving a child through artificial insemination can reasonably be regarded as a private action comparable to other interventions such as birth control and genetic screening, and perhaps no different from the supremely personal evolutionary decisions that any man and woman make when they marry and have children. Sperm-banking may remain a private matter in the United States, but you may be sure that more highly organized eugenic/reproductive agendas will emerge in the near future. What will we do when the first national leader announces a program to breed superior citizens? At what level are such issues to be dealt with? What kind of an international institutional framework—or political culture—might be necessary in order for discussion of such issues to take place?

It is easy enough to construct scenarios of biological developments that confound existing institutions of governance—much easier than to know what to do about them. The tempting response is to head all problems off at the pass: Outlaw genetic technology, outlaw artificial insemination or in vitro fertilization. This is not a very good solution—certainly not one that can be promiscuously applied.

That is what *cannot* be done. We don't know how to slow the general rate of change, apply the brakes to history, nip the Biological Revolution in the bud. It is the combined product of many lines of activity and the result of thousands of years of evolution, and no institution of governance has the power to halt forces of that magnitude. This is not to say that the Biological Revolution is beyond public control, that nothing can be done in the political realm to affect it. Quite the contrary: It vastly increases the range of social options and opens up whole new regions of public policy. There are countless ways public agencies can regulate it and influence its priorities. This will provide full employment for legislators and bureaucrats and diplomats, and draw upon the energies of political activists, for centuries to come.

The political activist needs to think not only about which issues of biopolitics to engage, but also about how to engage them. This is what I mean by a new *mode* of action. In the 1960s a certain kind of political activism—militant protest—caught the world's imagination, and as that particular chapter of history drew to a close it came to be widely believed that we were moving into a less political stage. In a certain sense we did—many people succumbed to the popular delusion that it is possible to be apolitical—but over the past couple of decades an entirely different wave of political activity has been gaining momentum. This is the activity connected with feedback, information gathering and distribution, global environmentalism; such work has been quietly preparing the way for entry into the most political era of all time. While we thought we were sinking into privatism we were in fact becoming ever more intimately connected to one another, citizens of the biosphere.

The appropriate political work of the time for many people will have to do with information. There will be legislative hearings, special commissions at all levels of government to take stock of current policies in such areas as species extinction, genetic resources, plant and animal movement, animal rights, human reproduction. There will be more scientific studies, more public conferences. Activists will have to deal with getting information and getting it to the right people. Organizations like the Worldwatch Institute have been doing the preparatory work for this new stage of politics, somewhat as the NAACP (with its patient labors that culminated in the *Brown v. Board of Education* decision in 1954) put down a foundation for an era of progress in civil rights.

We must not only recognize the important part played by information issues and information organizations, but adopt a style of political action grounded in the use of information—deliberately learning while acting, modifying course in response to feedback, knowing that there are risks and uncertainties in *all* courses of action.

I described the global restoration project as also a global learning project. There is really no other way to go at it: We have not, after all, done such a thing before. We can be sure that mistakes will be made, that some efforts will produce undesirable results and, quite possibly, problems as bad as those they were designed to solve. At the same time, we cannot decide not to proceed.

People who go into the trenches with restoration and development work, especially the kind based on communication between industrialized civilizations and primitive cultures—the work generally called "technology transfer"—have to steer a course between two dangers. One is the assumption that the local people merely need to be taught better ways of doing things—i.e., our ways. We have seen the evidence of that kind of shortcoming. On the other hand is the romantic notion that the people know what is to be done. This can be just as arrogant and just as mistaken. Peoples who have lived for centuries in a certain relationship to their environment know that way of life and that environment—but may know very little about other ways or understand how their environment is changing. The helper becomes a co-discoverer whose task is very similar to what some social scientists call "action research"—where information is intended not for learned journals, but for the people in the communities where it is obtained.

The learning dimension goes well beyond the merely technical aspects. There is also the deeper quest, the search for understanding of ourselves. Mythology and the arts and depth psychology remind us that when we embark upon such quests, we change. Each evolutionary project yields not only promises and problems, but meaning.

As species extinction becomes a political concern, those who take an interest in it are drawn into controversies about how a species is best protected, what a species *is*, what an ecosystem is—and beyond that into questions about why we should protect endangered species, what sort of relationship exists between humanity and the rest of earthly life that makes it either morally obligatory or economically expedient. Genetic erosion produces a similar mix of technical learning with consciousness-raising as people recognize the value of genetic resources and become aware of the global connections they create. Americans discover that their country is not only a breadbasket but also a gigantic surrogate mother to the germplasm from all over the world that is the progenitor of its herds and harvests.

Population is arguably the predominant global issue of our time, connected with all of the other questions that arise in the context of world politics. Few things could do more to ease the pressure on the world than a quick drop in the human birth rate. Such a change is certainly possible if the political energy for it existed, and there is no issue more accessible to us. And it is another of those political matters that is not merely a problem to be solved; it is a global schoolhouse about our species self-interest, our place in the biosphere. In the new mode of politics information and meaning are not a by-product, bringing some lesson to be ruefully learned along the way, but an integral part of all action.

The search for the shape of evolutionary politics brings a three-part discovery, then: a new framework of governance, a new content of issues, and a new mode of action. The framework is expansive and inclusive, and continually changing. The content is biopolitics—both the accumulated heritage of old interventions long ignored, and the surprising products of a scientific and technological revolution. The mode mixes action with thought, draws us into inquiry and philosophy even as we deal with fast-moving problems that seem to permit no time for reflection.

Another way to understand the political reality of our time is to consider the variety of possible near-term future developments. We have plenty of scenarios of problems and disasters, and equally plausible scenarios of great accomplishments. The answer to the question of what is to be done will increasingly be: Whatever we want to do. There are indeed limits but there is also room, as there has never been before, for utopian possibilities and grandiose agendas.

We have, for the first time in history, a surplus of options.

This signifies a great breakthrough in human evolution— one we have not really yet grasped—and it also presents a problem. Institutions of governance will have to be prepared to deal—on a more or less daily basis—with proposals and projects on a grand scale: California has to accomodate an organization that is breeding superior human beings, the Food and Agriculture Organization has to work out a system for global management of genetic resources. These are greater concerns than the institutions were designed to cope with; they point to the need for appropriate forms of governance, and for a cultural context within which we can deliberate projects concerning the human future, all earthly life, the biosphere itself.

Whichever way we turn, we are confronted with the prospect of human volition as a major determining force in the future of the Earth. Psychology and ecology overlap as we pursue the whys and hows of any issue. It becomes increasingly clear that the future of the biosphere is inseparable from the future of the human mind—that the destiny of every species and every ecosystem depends on what kind of progress is made in the realm of human thought and action. This is true regardless of what hopes one might have for the future. If we want a world of abundant wildlife and vast wilderness spaces and human-scale cities—a vision that I find immensely compelling—it is not to be achieved by backing away from the reality of our intervention, but by recognizing the full extent of it and going forward through new acts of imagination and creativity.

These considerations lead toward a different idea of the human species, and of each of us individually. Two thousand years ago Aristotle said that the human being is the political animal, which becomes what it is capable of being in the context of the polis. Today we begin to see that the human individual can only function, can only understand itself, can only be what it is, in the context of the larger polis which is the evolving biosphere.

This is neither an abstraction nor something yet to come about, but the present reality of everyday life. The steady trend of history has been toward the creation of artificial environments: cities, cultivated farms, managed wilderness areas, constructed waterways, and now reconstructed natural ecosystems. As our environments become more artificial, we live through new patterns of interaction that are unavoidably political. The same process that causes what I have called an escalation of intentionality also causes a collapse of privatism. Not only do boundaries between nations mean less, but so do boundaries between ecosystems and cultures—and so does the distance between the individual and the biosphere.

The basic truth about life in an artificial ecosystem can be discovered easily enough—it begins with a little reflection and research into the sources of one's air and water, food and medicine. The larger truth about one's personal citizenship in the biosphere—the truth summarized a few years ago in the title of Theodore Roszak's book *Person/ Planet*—will take longer to become a part of our political culture, and along the way it will come up hard against both the individualism of America and the collectivism of societies that have other ideas of what a person is a part of. But the truth is available because the postmodern world is all around us and within us, and the knowledge of how it works is there to be discovered in the homely reality of how we function as living organisms. And when that is comprehended none of us will have to search far to find a cause.

[Notes]

CHAPTER 1

1. Paul Tillich, A HISTORY OF CHRISTIAN THOUGHT (New York: Simon and Schuster, 1967), pp. 154–155.
2. (Pacific Palisades, Ca.: Goodyear [Prentice-Hall], 1976).
3. Most of the environmental modifications mentioned here are discussed at greater length in Raymond F. Dasmann, THE DESTRUCTION OF CALIFORNIA (New York: Collier Books, 1966).
4. Quoted in Paul and Anne Ehrlich, EXTINCTION (New York: Random House, 1981), p. 7.

CHAPTER 2

1. Samuel Butler, EREWHON (New York: E. P. Dutton, 1920), pp. 191–192.
2. Abraham Maslow, TOWARD A PSYCHOLOGY OF BEING (New York: Van Nostrand, 1962), p. 58.
3. George Gaylord Simpson, THE MEANING OF EVOLUTION, rev. ed. (New Haven: Yale University Press, 1967), pp. 286–287.
4. Omer C. Stewart, "Fire as the First Great Force Employed by Man," in William L. Thomas Jr. (ed), MAN'S ROLE IN CHANGING THE FACE OF THE EARTH (Chicago: University of Chicago Press, 1956), vol. 1, pp. 115 ff.; Ritchie Calder, AFTER THE SEVENTH DAY (New York: Simon and Schuster, 1961), p. 80.
5. J.A. Lauwerys, MAN'S IMPACT ON NATURE, (New York: Natural History Press, 1970), p. 48.
6. Karl A. Wittfogel, "The Hydraulic Civilizations," in Thomas, op. cit., pp. 152–164.

7. Lewis Mumford, "The Natural History of Urbanization," in Thomas, op. cit., pp. 382–398; see also Mumford, THE CITY IN HISTORY (New York: Harcourt, Brace & World, 1961).
8. Ritual regicide is one of the central themes of James G. Frazer, THE GOLDEN BOUGH (London: Macmillan, 1926). It is given fictional treatment in Mary Renault, THE KING MUST DIE (New York: Pantheon, 1958).
9. Aeschylus, "Prometheus Bound," in Edith Hamilton (trans.) THREE GREEK PLAYS (New York: Norton, 1937), p 115.
10. Aristotle, POLITICS, Book 1, Chapter 3.
11. Arthur Lovejoy, THE GREAT CHAIN OF BEING (Cambridge: Harvard University Press, 1953), p. 329.
12. Abbe Pluché, HISTOIRE DU CIEL, (1759 ed.), II, 391–392, quoted in Lovejoy, op. cit., p. 243.
13. Alexander Pope, "Essay On Man," in COMPLETE POETICAL WORKS (Boston: Houghton Mifflin, 1903), p. 192.
14. Soame Jenyns, NATURE AND ORIGIN OF EVIL (1757), 124–126, quoted in Lovejoy, op. cit., p. 203.
15. François Fénelon, TREATISE ON THE EXISTENCE OF GOD, I, 2, quoted in Lovejoy, op. cit., p. 186.
16. Robert Nisbet, HISTORY OF THE IDEA OF PROGRESS (New York: Basic Books, 1980), pp. 6–7.
17. Gottfried von Leibnitz, "On The Ultimate Origination of Things,"in Robert Latta (trans.) THE MONADOLOGY AND OTHER PHILOSOPHICAL WRITINGS (London: Oxford University Press, 1925), p. 350.
18. Condorcet, SKETCH FOR AN HISTORICAL PICTURE OF THE PROGRESS OF THE HUMAN MIND (1795), quoted in Nisbet, op. cit., pp. 210–211.
19. Buffon, "Epochs of Nature," in A NATURAL HISTORY, GENERAL AND PARTICULAR, trans. William Mellie, 2 vols. (London: Thomas Kelley & Co., 1866). See Clarence J. Glacken, "Changing Ideas of the Habitable World," in Thomas, op. cit., pp. 70–92.
20. See Steven M. Stanley, THE NEW EVOLUTIONARY TIMETABLE (Basic Books, 1981), p. 199.
21. Charles Darwin, THE ORIGIN OF SPECIES (New York: Mentor, 1958), p. 29.
22. Gertrude Himmelfarb, DARWIN AND THE DARWINIAN REVOLUTION (New York: Doubleday, 1959), p. 422.
23. Samuel Butler, LUCK OR CUNNING (London: Trubner, 1887), p. 291.

24. Himmelfarb, op. cit., p. 423.
25. Julian Huxley, introduction to Mentor edition, p. xv.
26. Darwin, op. cit., p. 69; see George Perkins Marsh, MAN AND NATURE (Cambridge: Harvard University Press, 1965), p. 247.
27. Herbert Spencer, SOCIAL STATICS (New York: Appleton, 1910); PRINCIPLES OF BIOLOGY (New York: Appleton, 1910), vol. 2, pp. 506–507.
28. William Graham Sumner, WHAT THE SOCIAL CLASSES OWE TO EACH OTHER (New York: Harper & Bros., 1883).
29. Marston Bates, "Man as an Agent in the Spread of Organisms," in Thomas, op. cit., p. 795.

CHAPTER 3

1. THE NEW EVOLUTIONARY TIMETABLE, p. 111.
2. Norman Myers, THE SINKING ARK (New York: Pergamon Press, 1979), p. 4.
3. EXTINCTION, p. 103ff.
4. Eward O. Wilson, BIOPHILIA (Cambridge: Harvard Univ. Press, 1984), p. 121.
5. Pat Roy Mooney, SEEDS OF THE EARTH (Ottawa: International Coalition for Development Action, 1979), p. 3.
6. J. B. Kendrick, Jr., "Preserving our Genetic Resources," CALIFORNIA AGRICULTURE, Sept. 1977, p. 2
7. Walt Reichert, "America's Diminishing Diversity," ENVIRONMENT, Nov. 1982, p. 8.
8. Carl L. Johannessen, "Domestication Process of Maize Continues in Guatemala," ECONOMIC BOTANY, Vol. 36 (1982), pp. 84–99.
9. SEEDS OF THE EARTH, p. 14.
10. Ken Conner, "Firms See Growth Potential in Seeds," *San Francisco Chronicle,* May 26, 1984, p. 48.
11. Jonathan King, "Patenting Modified Life Forms: The Case Against," *Environment,* July-August 1982, p. 40.
12. Mooney, THE LAW OF THE SEED (Uppsala: Dag Hammarskold Foundation, 1983), p. 13.
13. Peter Carlson, quoted in Steven C. Witt, BIOTECHNOLOGY AND GENETIC DIVERSITY (San Francisco: California Agricultural Lands Project, 1985), p. 69.
14. Jack Doyle, ALTERED HARVEST (N.Y.: Viking, 1985), p. 160.
15. J. R. Harlan, "The Green Revolution: Genetic Backlash," *Ceres— The Fao Review,* September-October 1969.

16. Recommended: Jeremy Cherfas, MAN-MADE LIFE (New York: Pantheon, 1982); Marc Lappé, BROKEN CODE (San Francisco: Sierra Club Books, 1985); Edward Yoxen, THE GENE BUSINESS (New York: Harper & Row, 1983); Burke K. Zimmerman, BIO-FUTURE (New York: Plenum, 1984).
17. THE GENE BUSINESS, p. 105.
18. MAN-MADE LIFE, p. 184.
19. Steven C. Witt, GENETIC ENGINEERING OF PLANTS (San Francisco: California Agricultural Lands Project, 1982), p. 43.
20. THE GENE BUSINESS, p. 130.
21. Noel Vietmeyer, "Exotic Edibles are Altering America's Diet and Agriculture," *Smithsonian*, December 1985, p. 37.
22. ALTERED HARVEST, p. 280.

CHAPTER 4

1. E.J. Hobsbawm, INDUSTRIAL EMPIRE: THE MAKING OF MODERN ENGLISH SOCIETY, Vol. II (New York: Pantheon, 1968), p. 1.
2. Karl Polanyi, THE GREAT TRANSFORMATION (Boston: Beacon Press, 1944), pp. 161–162.
3. Kerry Gruson, "Plight of an All-Male Species," *San Francisco Chronicle, This World*, Sept. 13, 1981, p. 25.
4. Phillip M. Hoose, BUILDING AN ARK (Covelo, CA: Island Press, 1981).
5. Norman Myers, A WEALTH OF WILD SPECIES (Boulder, CO: Westview Press, 1983).
6. Norman Myers, THE SINKING ARK (New York: Pergamon Press, 1979); Phillip M. Hoose, BUILDING AN ARK; Paul Ehrlich and Dennis C. Pirages, ARK II: A SOCIAL RESPONSE TO ENVIRONMENTAL IMPERATIVES; re the "Noah principle," see David Ehrenfeld, THE ARROGANCE OF HUMANISM (Oxford, 1978).
7. Jack Doyle, ALTERED HARVEST (New York: Viking, 1985), p. 13.
8. Earl L. Green, "Maintenance and Breeding of Genetic Stocks of Mice for Research," PROCEEDINGS, SYMPOSIUM AND WORKSHOP ON GENETIC RESOURCES CONSERVATION FOR CALIFORNIA, sponsored by the University of California, Division of Agriculture and Natural Resources, and The California Department of Food and Agriculture, Napa, CA., April 5–7, 1984, p. 9.

9. D. L. Plucknett et al., "Crop Germplasm Conservation and Developing Countries," *Science*, April 8, 1983, pp. 163–169.

10. M. S. Swaminathan, "Genetic Conservation—Microbes to Man," *Genetic Engineering and Biotechnology Monitor* (Vienna, Austria: United Nations Industrial Development Organization), Issue No. 8 (1984), p. 71.

11. Pat Roy Mooney, THE LAW OF THE SEED: ANOTHER DEVELOPMENT AND PLANT GENETIC RESOURCES (Uppsala, Sweden: The Dag Hammarskjold Centre, 1983), p. 29.

12. I have referred to all forms of plant right protection as "patenting." Actually, the 1930 Plant Patent Act extended patent protection to certain plant varieties, while the later Plant Variety Protection Act set up a separate "patent-like" protection administered by USDA.

13. Tamar Lewin, "Genetic Engineering: To Patent Everything in Sight?" *Technology Review*, Feb./March 1983, p. 33.

14. LAW OF THE SEED, p. 154.

15. Edward Yoxen, THE GENE BUSINESS, p. 22.

16. Burke K. Zimmerman, BIOFUTURE, p. 103.

17. *Diamond v. Chakrabarty et al.*, no. 79–136, June 16, 1980.

18. THE GENE BUSINESS, p. 93.

19. H. C. Trowell and D. P. Burkitt (eds), WESTERN DISEASES: THEIR EMERGENCE AND PREVENTION (London: Edward Arnold, 1981).

20. BROKEN CODE, pp. 80–81.

21. ALTERED HARVEST, p. 86.

22. Bill Soiffer, "An 'Explosion' of Big-Money Lawsuits on Toxic Pollution," *San Francisco Chronicle*, July 5, 1985, p. 4.

23. ALTERED HARVEST, p. 224.

24. BIOFUTURE, p. 137.

25. BIOFUTURE, p. 142.

26. THE GENE BUSINESS, p. 48.

27. Liebe Cavalieri, "New Strains of Life—Or Death," *New York Times Magazine*, August 22, 1976, p. 8.

28. BIOFUTURE, p. 171.

29. *Genetic Engineering and Biotechnology Monitor*, Issue 6 (1983), p. 8.

30. *Genetic Engineering and Biotechnology Monitor*, Issue 6, p. 9.

31. Philip M. Boffey, "The Risks of Biological Roulette," *San Francisco Chronicle, This World*, Sept. 30, 1984, pp. 16–17.

32. Gar Smith, "Man-made Bacteria Halted in the Fields; Secretly Released in Oakland," *Earth Island Journal*, March 1986, p. 4.

33. Richard Saltus, "Ban urged on genetic experiments to create super animals," *San Francisco Examiner*, Sept. 30, 1984, p. A8.

34. BROKEN CODE, p.270.
35. John Elkington, THE GENE FACTORY (New York: Carroll & Graf), 1985, p. 98.
36. BROKEN CODE, P. 250.
37. BROKEN CODE, p. 237.
38. BIOFUTURE, p. 142.
39. Gena Kolata, "How Safe Are Engineered Organisms?" *Science*, July 5, 1984, p. 35.
40. Paul and Anne Ehrlich, EXTINCTION, p. 121.
41. James Coates, "Foreigners accused of massive plunder of U. S. wildlife," *San Francisco Chronicle*, Oct. 14, 1984, p. A16.
42. EXTINCTION, p. 122.
43. Peter Raven, "Disappearing Species: A Global Tragedy," *The Futurist*, Oct. 1985, p. 14.
44. See Hoose, BUILDING AN ARK.
45. State of California, Assembly Office of Research, "Review of Federal and State Regulations Affecting the California Biotechnology Industry," 1985.
46. Barry Commoner, "The Politics of Biotechnology," public lecture, Marin Community College, Kentfield, California, Dec. 4, 1984.
47. Gordon Orions, quoted in Roger Lewin, "Why Dynamiting Vampire Bats Is Wrong," *Science*, April 4, 1986, p. 24. The report cited is ECOLOGICAL KNOWLEDGE AND ENVIRONMENTAL PROBLEM-SOLVING (Washington, D.C.: National Academy Press, 1986).

CHAPTER 5

1. Francis Galton, HEREDITARY GENIUS (London: Julian Friedmann, 1979).
2. Daniel J. Kevles, "Annals of Eugenics," Part I, *The New Yorker*, Oct. 8, 1984, p. 51. These articles have been published in book form as IN THE NAME OF EUGENICS (New York: Knopf, 1985).
3. Kevles, p. 102.
4. Kevles, p. 104.
5. Kevles, p. 102.
6. Marc Lappé, GENETIC POLITICS: THE LIMITS OF BIOLOGICAL CONTROL (New York: Simon and Schuster, 1979), p. 18.
7. GENETIC POLITICS, p. 89.
8. GENETIC POLITICS, p. 18.

9. GENETIC POLITICS, p. 19.
10. Frederick Ausubel, Jon Beckwith, and Kaaren Janssen, "The Politics of Genetic Engineering," *Psychology Today*, June 1974, p. 40.
11. Kevles, Part II, Oct. 15, 1984, p. 125.
12. Kevles, Part II, p. 113.
13. Kevles, Part III, Oct. 22, 1984, p. 144.
14. Walter Laquer, THE TERRIBLE SECRET (Boston: Little, Brown, 1980.)
15. Sheldon C. Reed, "History of Genetic Counseling," *Social Biology* 21:332 (1974).
16. Philip Reilly, GENETICS, LAW AND SOCIAL POLICY (Cambridge: Harvard University Press, 1977), p. 46.
17. Kevles, Part IV, Oct. 29, 1984, p. 87.
18. GENETIC POLITICS, p. 97.
19. Gina Kolata, "Genetic Screening Raises Questions for Employers and Insurers," *Science*, April 18, 1986, p. 317.
20. Morton Hunt, "The Total Gene Screen," *New York Times Magazine*, Jan. 19, 1986, p. 38.
21. D. Rorvik, "The Embryo Sweepstakes", *New York Times Magazine*, September 15, 1974, p. 17.
22. Claudia Wallis, "A Surrogate's Story," *Time*, September 10, 1984, p. 53.
23. Fern Schumer Chapman, "Going for Gold in the Baby Business," *Fortune*, Sept. 17, 1984, p. 47.
24. Otto Friedrich, "A Legal, Moral, Social Nighmare," *Time*, Sept. 10, 1984, p. 54.
25. Gena Corea, THE MOTHER MACHINE (New York: Harper & Row, 1985), pp. 4–8.
26. Jeff Lyon, PLAYING GOD IN THE NURSERY (New York: Norton, 1985), pp. 24–25.
27. "Baby Jane Doe at Stony Brook: A Chronology," background paper, conference on Treatment of Handicapped Newborns: Medical, Ethical and Social Issues, State University of New York at Stony Brook, October 17–20, 1984.
28. John Lorber, "The Doctor's Duty to Patients and Parents in Profoundly Handicapped Conditions," paper presented at symposium, Center for Bioethics, Clinical Research Insitute of Montreal, Montreal, Quebec, Canada, November 18, 1976.
29. Shulamith Firestone, THE DIALECTIC OF SEX (New York: William Morrow, 1976), p. 270.
30. Peter Singer and Deane Wells, MAKING BABIES (New York: Scribner's, 1985), p. 119.

31. GENETICS, LAW AND SOCIAL POLICY, p. 199.
32. David Perlman, "Fertilization Specialists Hail Saving of Orphan Embryos," *San Francisco Chronicle*, Oct. 25, 1984, p. 9.
33. Friedrich, p. 55.
34. Friedrich, p. 54.
35. Aldous Huxley, BRAVE NEW WORLD REVISITED (New York: Harper & Row, 1965), pp. 11–12.
36. Kevles, Part IV, p. 109.
37. Kevles, Part IV, p. 98.
38. GENETICS, LAW AND SOCIAL POLICY, p. 143.
39. K. Kondo and T. Tsubaki, "Abortion Programme in Duchenne Muscular Dystrophy in Japan," *Lancet*, 1:543 (1973).
40. Kevles, Part IV, p. 60.
41. Kevles, Part IV, p. 90.
42. Kevles, Part IV, p. 90.
43. GENETICS, LAW AND SOCIAL POLICY, p. 205.
44. Friedrich, p. 56.
45. HEREDITARY GENIUS, p. x.
46. Stephen Jay Gould, THE MISMEASURE OF MAN (New York: Norton, 1981), p. 146.
47. THE MISMEASURE OF MAN, p. 163.
48. Cyril Burt, "The Inheritance of General Intelligence," *American Psychology*, 1972, 27, p. 188.
49. THE MISMEASURE OF MAN, p. 235.
50. GENETICS, LAW AND SOCIAL POLICY, p. 240.
51. GENETIC POLITICS, p. 92.
52. Thomas Malthus, ON POPULATION (New York: Mentor, 1960), p. 57.
53. Paul Ehrlich, THE POPULATION BOMB (New York: Ballantine, 1968), p. 4.
54. Pranay Gupte, THE CROWDED EARTH (New York: Norton, 1984), p. 31.
55. Lester R. Brown et al., STATE OF THE WORLD 1984 (New York: Norton, 1984), p. 24.
56. THE CROWDED EARTH, p. 38.
57. THE CROWDED EARTH, p. 188, p. 303.
58. Julian L. Simon, THE ULTIMATE RESOURCE (Princeton: Princeton University Press, 1981), p. 192.
59. THE CROWDED EARTH, p. 20.
60. Garrett Hardin, "The Tragedy of the Commons," in Garrett De Bell (ed.), THE ENVIRONMENTAL HANDBOOK (New York: Ballantine, 1970), p. 42.

61. "Beyond Environmentalism: The Biological Foundations of Governance," in Anderson (ed.), RETHINKING LIBERALISM (New York: Avon, 1983), p. 248.

CHAPTER 6

1. Peter Singer, ANIMAL LIBERATION: A NEW ETHICS FOR OUR TREATMENT OF ANIMALS (New York: Avon, 1975), p. 1.
2. Frederick Pohl and C. M. Kornbluth, THE SPACE MERCHANTS (New York: Ballantine, 1953).
3. Information provided by The Humane Society of the United States, Washington, D.C.
4. Singer, p. 31.
5. U. S. Congress, Office of Technology Assessment, ALTERNATIVES TO ANIMAL USE IN RESEARCH, TESTING AND EDUCATION (Washington, D.C.: U. S. Government Printing Office, Feb. 1986.)
6. Bernard E. Rollin, ANIMAL RIGHTS AND HUMAN MORALITY (Buffalo, N.Y.: Prometheus, 1981), p. 91.
7. Windeatt and May, "Charles River: The General Motors of Animal Breeding," The Beast, Summer 1980, p. 27.
8. Singer, p. 43.
9. Douglas Starr, "Equal Rights," Audubon, November 1984, p. 30.
10. Michael D. Ware, "The ALF Strikes," Agenda (News Magazine of the Animal Rights Network), July/August 1984, p. 8.
11. Jim Mason, "Animal Rights," The Utne Reader, Dec. 1984/Jan. 1985, pp. 22–23.
12. Don W. Allen, "The Rights of Nonhuman Animals and World Public Order: A Global Assessment," New York Law School Law Review, Vol. 28 (1983), p. 408.
13. Jim Mason, "Prominent Scientist Convicted—Animal Cruelty Clears a Major Legal Hurdle," Pacific News Service, 604 Mission St., San Francisco CA 94105.
14. PETA News (undated), People for the Ethical Treatment of Animals, P. O. Box 42516, Washington, D.C. 20015.
15. ANIMAL RIGHTS: WHAT'S IT ALL ABOUT?, Trans-Species Unlimited, P.O. Box 1351, State College PA 16804.
16. Rollin, p. 5.
17. Ronald W. Clark, THE SURVIVAL OF CHARLES DARWIN (New York: Random House, 1985), p. 76.

18. Singer, ANIMAL LIBERATION, pp. 8–9.
19. Tom Regan, THE CASE FOR ANIMAL RIGHTS (Berkeley: University of California Press, 1983), p. 329.
20. Michael Allen Fox, THE CASE FOR ANIMAL EXPERIMENTATION (Berkeley: University of California Press, 1986), p. 50.
21. Allen, p. 423.
22. Allen, p. 402.
23. Christopher Stone, SHOULD TREES HAVE STANDING? (Los Altos, CA: William Kaufmann, 1974), p. 17.
24. *Palila v. Hawaii Dep't of Land & Natural Resources*, 471 F. Supp. 985.
25. William Kahrl, "Animal rights: a mistaken priority?" *Oakland Tribune*, Feb. 6, 1985.
26. Mark Dowie, "Looking for the Right Animal Story," *Insider*, Winter 1985, p. 1.
27. Burke Zimmerman, comments at "Just Like Us?—Debate on Animal Rights," College of Marin, Feb. 26, 1986, sponsored by Foundation for Ethical Studies, 350 Starling Road, Mill Valley CA 94941.
28. U. S. Congress, Office of Technology Assessment, *op. cit.*
29. Quoted in Frances Moore Lappé, DIET FOR A SMALL PLANET, (New York: Ballantine, 1975), p. 43.

CHAPTER 7

1. On nitrogen compounds: Bert Bolin and Erik Arrhenius (eds.), "Nitrogen—An Essential Life Factor and a Growing Environmental Hazard: Report from Nobel Symposium No. 38," *Ambio,* Number 2–3, 1977. On acid pollution: John McCormick, ACID EARTH (London: Earthscan, 1985).
2. George Perkins Marsh, MAN AND NATURE, OR, PHYSICAL GEOGRAPHY AS MODIFIED BY HUMAN ACTION (Cambridge: Harvard University Press, 1965 [first published 1864]).
3. Lynton K. Caldwell has done extensive research on the origins of this word. See his INTERNATIONAL ENVIRONMENTAL POLICY (Durham, N. C.: Duke University Press, 1984), p. 21ff., and Caldwell, IN DEFENSE OF EARTH: INTERNATIONAL PROTECTION OF THE BIOSPHERE (Bloomington: Indiana University Press, 1972), Ch. 2; and G. Evelyn Hutchinson, "The Biosphere," *Scientific American*), Sept. 1970, p. 45. I am indebted to Prof. Caldwell for the phrase "discovery of the biosphere," which was first used by him in IN DEFENSE OF EARTH.

Notes

4. V. I. Vernadsky, "The Biosphere and the Noosphere," *American Scientist*, Jan. 1945, p. 4.
5. Julian Huxley, introduction to Pierre Teilhard de Chardin, THE PHENOMENON OF MAN (New York: Harper & Brothers, 1959), p. 13.
6. Vernadsky, p. 9.
7. William L. Thomas, Jr. (ed.), MAN'S ROLE IN CHANGING THE FACE OF THE EARTH (Chicago: University of Chicago Press, 1956).
8. Caldwell, INTERNATIONAL ENVIRONMENTAL POLICY, p. 25.
9. UNESCO, "Final Report on the Biosphere."
10. Maurice Strong, "One Year After Stockholm: An Ecological Approach to Management," *Foreign Affairs*, July 1973, p. 261.
11. Caldwell, INTERNATIONAL ENVIRONMENTAL POLICY, p. 53.
12. Gary W. Barrett, "A Problem-Solving Approach to Resource Management," *BioScience*, July/August 1985, pp. 423–427.
13. Donella H. Meadows et al, THE LIMITS TO GROWTH (New York: New American Library, 1972).
14. THE GLOBAL 2000 REPORT TO THE PRESIDENT (New York: Penguin, 1982), pp. 1–4.
15. Herman Kahn and Julian Simon (eds.) THE RESOURCEFUL EARTH; A RESPONSE TO GLOBAL 2000 (New York: Basil Blackwell, 1984).
16. Edward O. Wilson, "The Biological Diversity Crisis," *BioScience*, December 1985, pp. 700–706.
17. Norman Myers (ed.), GAIA: AN ATLAS OF PLANET MANAGEMENT (Garden City, N.Y.: Anchor, 1984), pp. 238–239.
18. John Kenneth Galbraith, THE NEW INDUSTRIAL STATE (Boston: Houghton Mifflin, 1971), p. 299.
19. Lee Kimball, "The Law of the Sea," *Environment*, November 1983, p. 14.
20. William Wertenbecker, "A Reporter at Large—Law of the Sea Conference," *The New Yorker*, August 1, 1983, p. 42.
21. Kimball, p. 41.

CHAPTER 8

1. Robert N. Bellah et al., HABITS OF THE HEART (Berkeley: University of California Press, 1985), p. 20.

2. Clyde Kluckhohn and William H. Kelly, "The Concept of Culture," in THE SCIENCE OF MAN IN THE WORLD CRISIS (New York: Columbia University Press, 1945), p. 91.
3. Kenneth E. Boulding, EVOLUTIONARY ECONOMICS (Beverly Hills: Sage, 1981), p. 16.
4. Joshua Meyrowitz, NO SENSE OF PLACE (New York: Oxford University Press, 1985), p. 8.
5. Susan Sontag, "Notes on 'Camp,'" in AGAINST INTERPRETATION (New York: Farrar, Straus & Giroux, 1966), pp. 275–292.
6. Lynn White, Jr., "The Historical Roots of our Ecologic Crisis," can be found in many collections of environmental writings including my own: POLITICS AND ENVIRONMENT (Pacific Palisades, CA: Goodyear [Prentice-Hall]), 1971; Second edition, 1975).
7. René Dubos, A GOD WITHIN (New York: Scribners, 1972), pp. 167, 174.
8. Alan W. Watts, "The Individual as Man/World," in POLITICS AND ENVIRONMENT.
9. Lynn White Jr. has likened the publication in English of D. T. Suzuki's essays on Zen to the publication of translations of Plato and Aristotle in pre-Renaissance Europe, and Arnold Toynbee has forecast a non-military conquest of the West by the East. See Houston Smith, introduction to Swami Pravhavananda, THE SPIRITUAL HERITAGE OF INDIA (Hollywood: Vedanta Press, 1963).
10. Jaroslav Pelikan, quoted in HABITS OF THE HEART, p. 140.
11. Lester Milbrath, ENVIRONMENTALISTS: VANGUARD FOR A NEW SOCIETY (Albany: State University of New York Press, 1984), p. 98.
12. Milbrath, p. 26.
13. Ernest Callenbach, ECOTOPIA (New York: Bantam, 1973).
14. Donald N. Michael, ON LEARNING TO PLAN—AND PLANNING TO LEARN (San Francisco: Jossey-Bass, 1973). Also see Michael, "Neither Hierarchy nor Anarchy: Notes on Norms for Governance in a Systemic World," in Anderson (ed.) RETHINKING LIBERALISM.
15. See Edward O. Wilson, SOCIOBIOLOGY: THE NEW SYNTHESIS (Cambridge: Harvard University Press, 1975); Arthur L. Caplan (ed.) THE SOCIOBIOLOGY DEBATE (New York: Harper & Row, 1978).
16. Melvin Konner, THE TANGLED WING (New York: Holt, Rinehart & Winston, 1982).

17. Ludwig von Bertalanffy, ROBOTS, MEN AND MINDS (New York: Braziller, 1967), pp. 34–35.
18. Roger D. Masters, "The Political Implications of Sociobiology, Part III: Birth Control, Celibacy, and Inclusive Fitness," paper presented at the Second Annual Meeting of the International Society of Political Psychology, Washington, D. C., 1981, p. 37.
19. Pico della Mirandola, "Oration on the Dignity of Man," quoted in Niccola Abbagnano, "Humanism," trans. Nino Langiulli, in Paul Edwards (ed.) ENCYCLOPEDIA OF PHILOSOPHY (New York: Macmillan, 1967), 4:70.

CHAPTER 9

1. GAIA: AN ATLAS OF PLANET MANAGEMENT, p. 14.
2. See Robert Heilbroner, THE ECONOMIC PROBLEM (Englewood Cliffs, N.J.: Prentice-Hall, 1972), pp. 570–571; and K. William Kapp, THE SOCIAL COSTS OF PRIVATE ENTERPRISE (Cambridge, Mass.: Harvard University Press, 1950).
3. Freud, CIVILIZATION AND ITS DISCONTENTS, trans. James Strachey (New York: Norton, 1962), p. 80.
4. Bill Devall and George Sessions, DEEP ECOLOGY (Salt Lake City: Peregrine Smith, 1985). The term "deep ecology" is the creation of the Norwegian philosopher Arne Naess.
5. Edward O. Wilson, BIOPHILIA (Harvard University Press, 1984).
6. Bill Devall, "Streams of Environmentalism," *Natural Resources Journal* (University of New Mexico School of Law), Spring 1979.
7. Edgar Z. Friedenberg, COMING OF AGE IN AMERICA (New York: Random House, 1965), pp. 47–48.
8. Rollo May, POWER AND INNOCENCE (New York: Norton, 1972) p. 53.
9. Hans Ruesch, SLAUGHTER OF THE INNOCENT (New York: Bantam, 1978).
10. Bill Soiffer, "Guerrillas in the War Over the Environment," *San Francisco Chronicle*, October 31, 1985, p. 40.
11. Jeremy Rifkin, DECLARATION OF A HERETIC (New York: Routledge & Kegan Paul, 1985).
12. John J. Berger, RESTORING THE EARTH (New York: Knopf, 1985).
13. Zhang Bihua, "Reclaiming the Land of Genghis Khan," 1984, Earthscan, 3 Endsleigh Street, London WC1H ODD.
14. John Todd, "The Ocean Pickup on the Spanish Main," *Annals of Earth Stewardship*, Vol. II, Number 2, 1984.

15. Peter Raven, "Global Futures: The Third World," paper presented to the American Association for the Advancement of Science, New York, May 25, 1984; Paulo Nogueira-Neto, "Getting Brazil's Network of Ecological Stations on the Ground," *Journal '85* (World Resources Institute).
16. See Richard Register, ANOTHER BEGINNING (Berkeley: Treehouse, 1978); and Nancy Jack Todd and John Todd, BIOSHELTERS, OCEAN ARKS, CITY FARMING (San Francisco: Sierra Club, 1984).
17. John J. Berger, "The Prairie Makers," *Sierra*, Nov. 1985, pp. 64–70.
18. Stephen Toulmin, THE RETURN TO COSMOLOGY (Berkeley: University of California Press, 1982), p. 254. (Italics in original.)
19. On the "new paradigm" perspective see Fritjof Capra, THE TURNING POINT (New York: Simon and Schuster, 1982). For a discussion of the "new environmental paradigm," see Lester Milbrath, ENVIRONMENTALISTS: VANGUARD FOR A NEW SOCIETY (Albany, NY: State University of New York Press, 1984.)
20. Peter A. Corning, THE SYNERGISM HYPOTHESIS (New York: McGraw-Hill, 1983).
21. See, for example, William Irwin Thompson, AT THE EDGE OF HISTORY (New York: Harper & Row, 1972); William R. Fix, THE BONE PEDDLERS (New York: Macmillan, 1984).